Pet owner educational atlas

CATS

SERVET

Plaza Antonio Beltrán Martínez nº 1, planta 8 - letra I
(Centro empresarial El Trovador)
50002 Zaragoza - Spain

First printing: August 2014

This book was originally published in Spanish under the title
Atlas de información al propietario. Especie Felina
© 2013 Grupo Asís Biomedia, SL
ISBN Spanish edition: 978-84-940402-0-7

Translation:
Melissa Testa

Illustrators:
Jacob Gragera Artal
Paula Marco Peinado

ISBN: 978-84-942829-2-8
DL: Z 1104-2014

Design, layout and printing:
Servet editorial - Grupo Asís Biomedia, SL
www.grupoasis.com
info@grupoasis.com

Servet is the publishing house of Grupo Asís

Warning:

Veterinary science is constantly evolving, as are pharmacology and the other sciences. Inevitably, it is therefore the responsibility of the veterinary surgeon to determine and verify the dosage, the method of administration, the duration of treatment and any possible contraindications to the treatments given to each individual patient, based on his or her professional experience. Neither the publisher nor the author can be held liable for any damage or harm caused to people, animals or properties resulting from the correct or incorrect application of the information contained in this book.

PROLOGUE

Why an atlas of procedures and diseases in cats? Images are always more powerful than words and on more than one occasion, I have thus found myself in the consultation room making drawings about diseases for owners eager to understand what was happening to their cat and what our treatment plan was. I therefore thought this project was truly interesting.

This atlas is the result of intensive work to gather diagnostic procedures, diseases organised by system and differential diagnoses shown by means of scientifically rigorous illustrations. All of them are based on recent studies in feline medicine, with the objective of providing all the necessary explanations to cat owners in a simple and practical manner.

It is of vital importance that cat owners understand the disease their animal is suffering from so they comply with our indications. If we stop to think about what owners feel like from the moment they place their cat in the carrier, until that when they chase the animal to administer a treatment they do not really know what it is for... we will understand why, on many occasions, compliance with treatments is low and, what is worse, why our patient is not taken to the veterinary practice.

If we can make owners understand why a treatment is necessary, they will do their best to comply with our guidelines and, what is more important, they will take their cats for regular check-ups to control their disease. That is why this new tool is essential in daily practice.

Mª Luisa Palmero
AVEPA Recognised Specialist in Feline Medicine
GPCert (FelP)
Gattos Feline Clinical Centre

Table of contents

Endocrine system

Skin and adnexa

Digestive system

Nervous system

Eyes

03 INFECTIOUS DISEASES

04 SPECIAL TECHNIQUES

05 BEHAVIOUR AND MANAGEMENT

1 Cat skeleton

Fibrous, cartilaginous and synovial joints

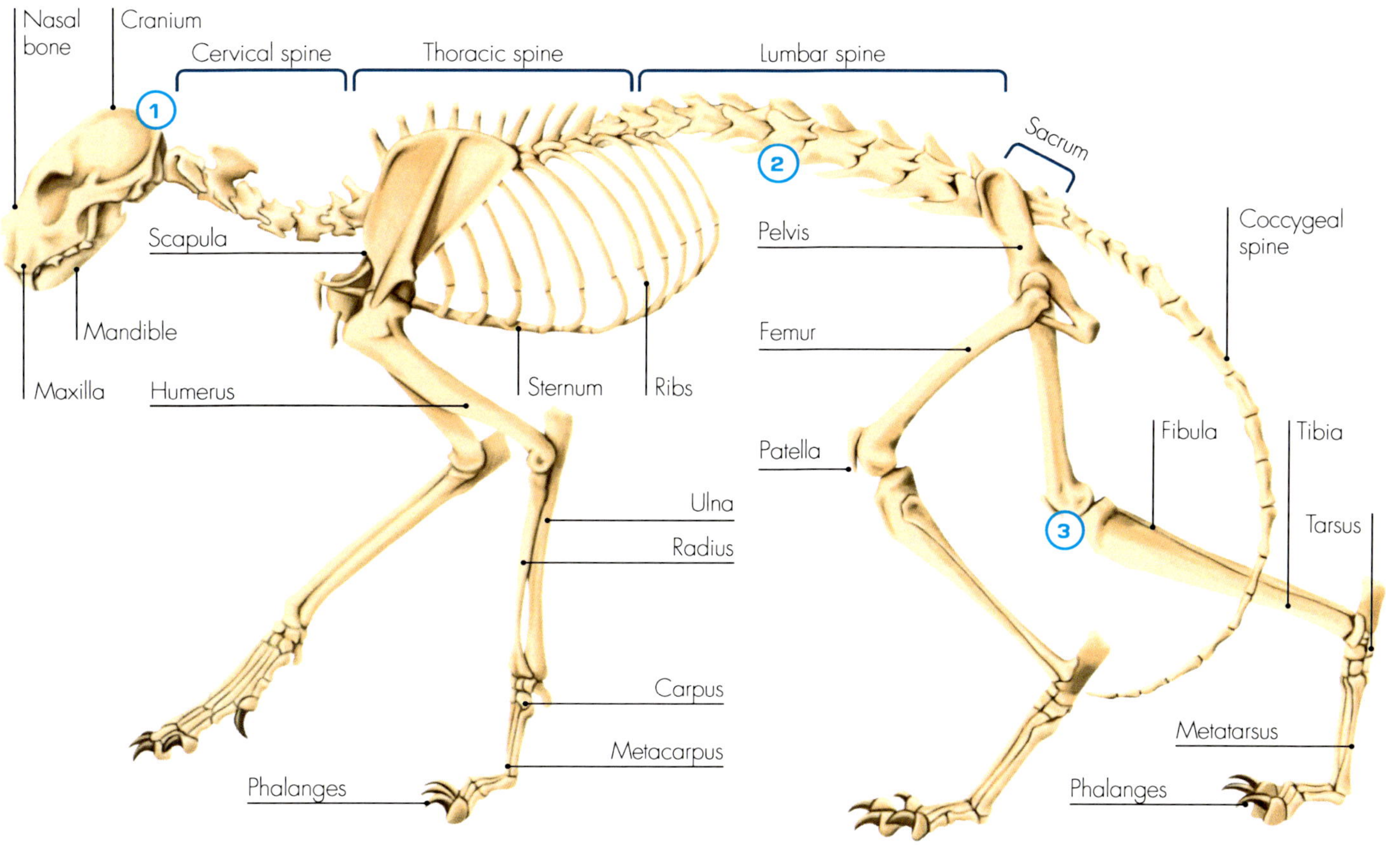

1 FIBROUS JOINT
(cranial sutures)

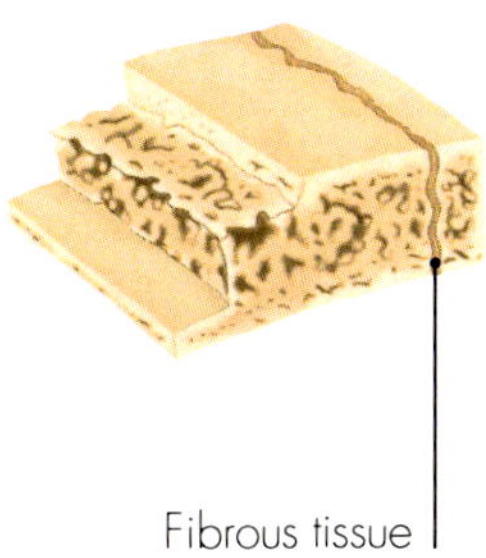

2 CARTILAGINOUS JOINT
(intervertebral joints)

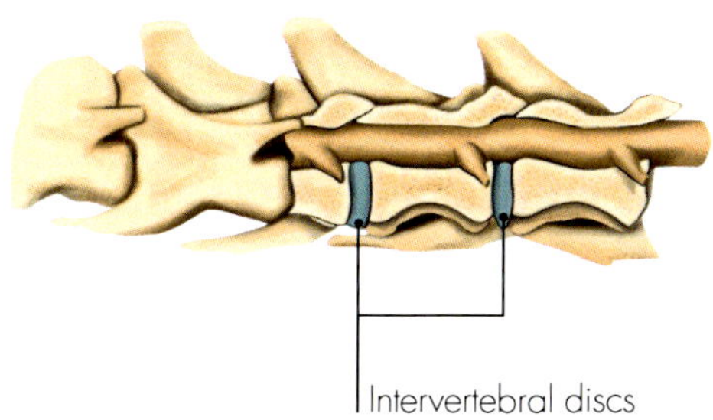

3 SYNOVIAL JOINT
(stifle, elbow, shoulder, hip, etc.)

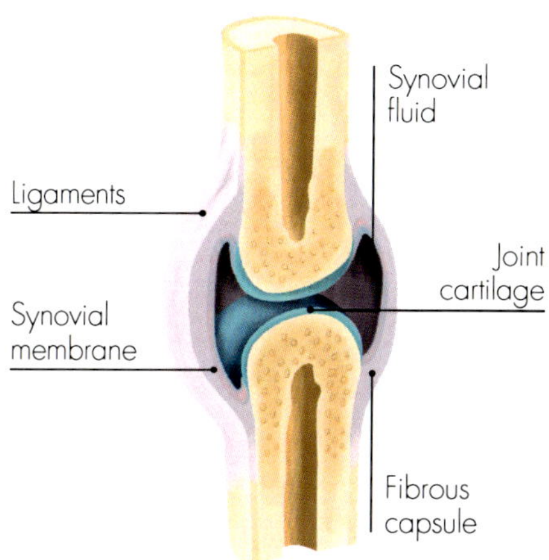

2 Cat muscles

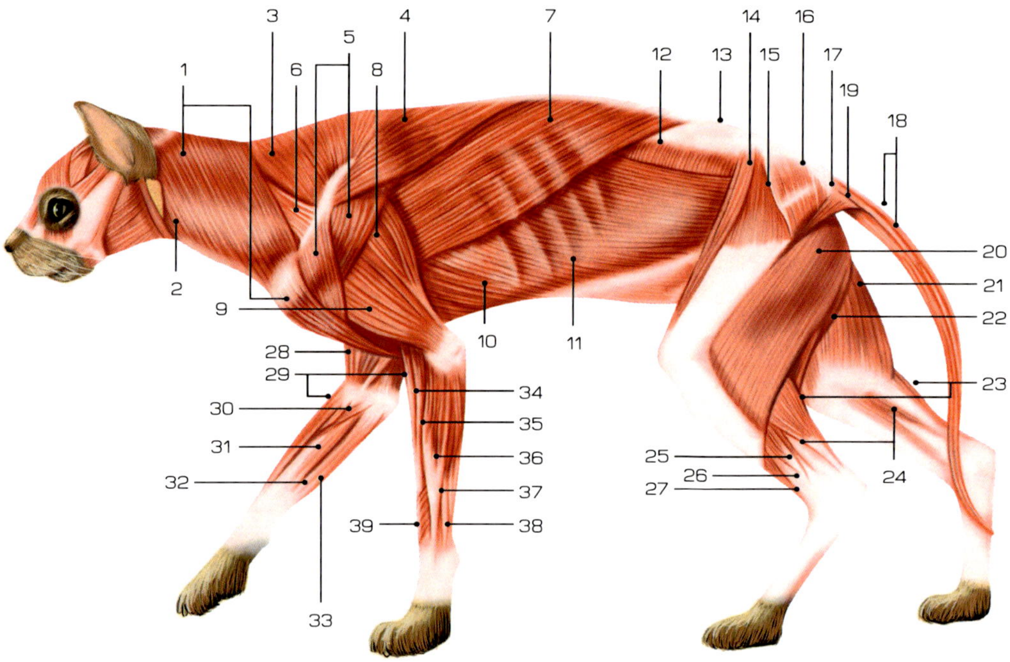

1. Brachiocephalic muscle (cleidocephalicus and cleidobrachialis)
2. Sternocephalic muscle
3. Trapezius muscle (cervical part)
4. Trapezius muscle (thoracic part)
5. Deltoid muscle
6. Omotransversarius muscle
7. Latissimus dorsi muscle
8. Triceps brachii muscle (long head)
9. Triceps brachii muscle (lateral head)
10. Deep pectoral muscle
11. Abdominal external oblique muscle
12. Abdominal internal oblique muscle
13. Thoracolumbar fascia
14. Sartorius muscle
15. Tensor fasciae latae muscle
16. Gluteus medius muscle
17. Gluteus superficialis muscle
18. Sacrocaudal muscles
19. Caudofemoralis muscles
20. Biceps femoris muscle
21. Semimembranosus muscle
22. Semitendinosus muscle
23. Gastrocnemius muscle
24. Deep digital flexor muscle
25. Lateral digital extensor muscle
26. Peroneus longus muscle
27. Tibialis cranialis muscle
28. Biceps brachii muscle
29. Brachioradialis muscle
30. Pronator teres muscle
31. Extensor carpi radialis muscle
32. Flexor carpi radialis muscle
33. Superficial digital flexor muscle
34. Extensor carpi radialis muscle
35. Extensor digitorum communis muscle
36. Extensor digitorum lateralis muscle
37. Extensor carpi ulnaris muscle
38. Flexor carpi ulnaris muscle
39. Digital abductor muscle

Muscles of the face

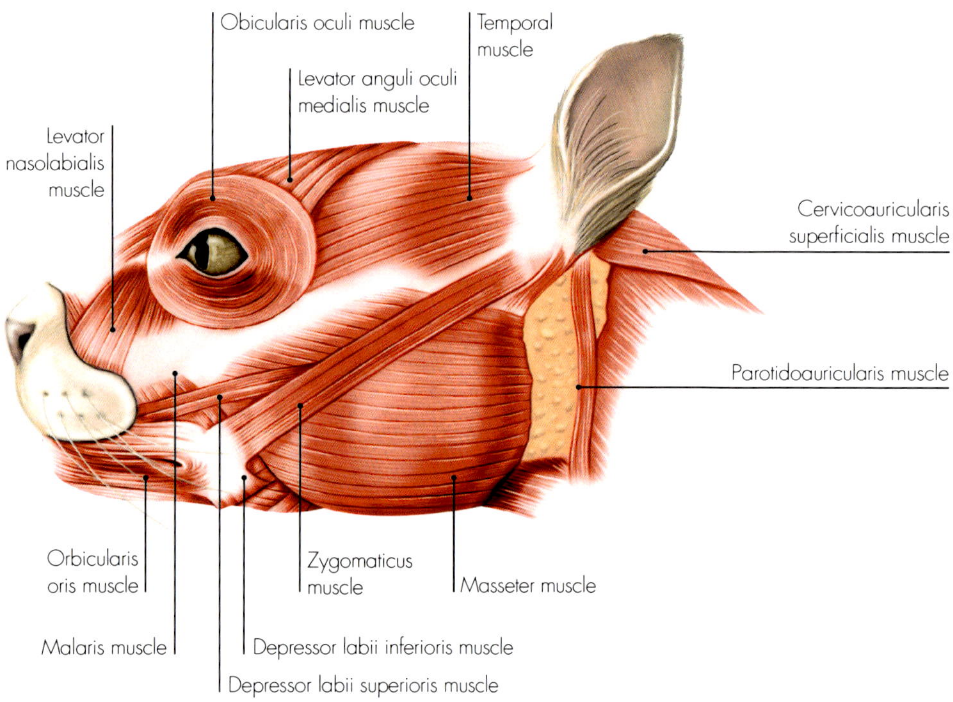

MUSCULOSKELETAL SYSTEM

3 Lesions of the mandible

Traumatic separation of the mandibular symphysis: repair by means of cerclage wire

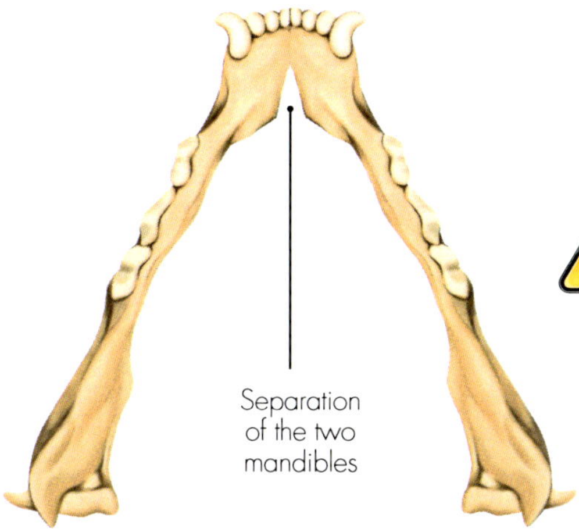

It may also be repaired by applying a splint from canine to canine with dentistry material.

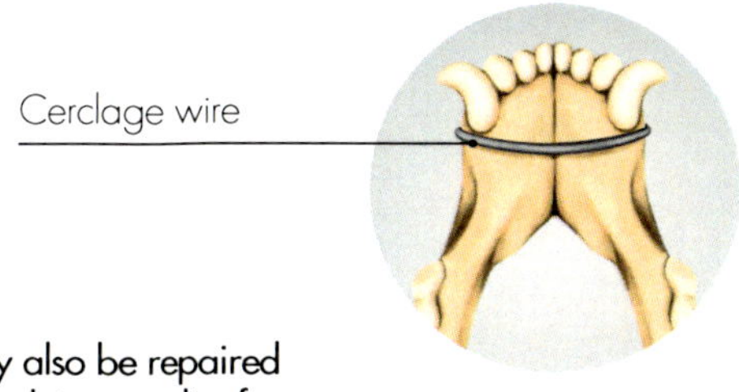

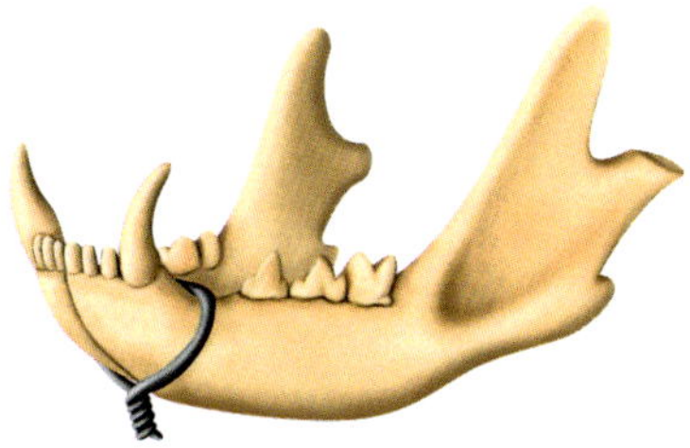

Temporomandibular joint luxation

Temporomandibular luxation is due to trauma (falls, road traffic accidents) and is almost always unilateral, although it may on occasions be bilateral. Luxation may be in a rostral dorsal or caudal ventral direction, the latter having a poorer prognosis as it is associated with fractures in the joint area.

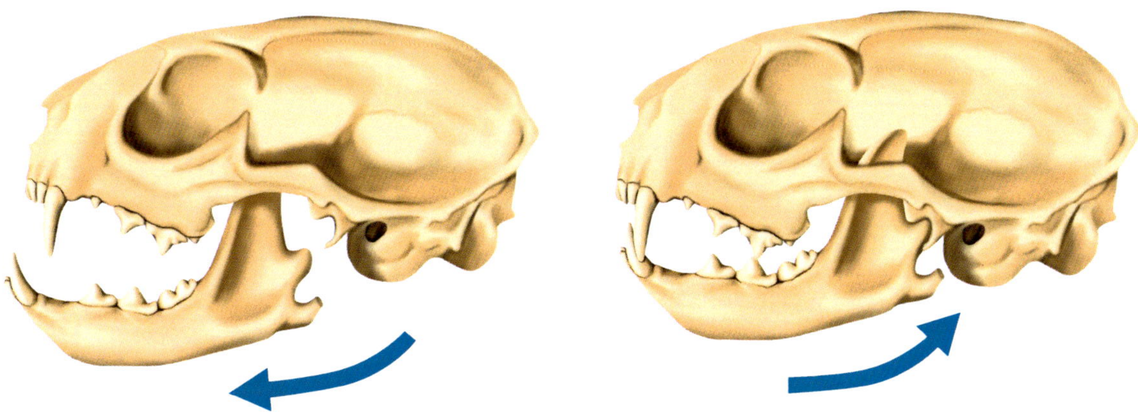

Medical treatment
Reduction of luxation and immobilisation of the area.

Surgical treatment
In cases in which the joint is fractured, due to the risk of ankylosis.

Clinical signs

- Dropped mandible and malocclusion.
- Inability to close the mouth.
- Hypersalivation.

MUSCULOSKELETAL SYSTEM

4 Osteoarthritis

Degenerative joint disease

Osteoarthritis may go unnoticed as its symptoms are attributed to age instead of joint pain. The most affected joints are the hip and the elbows, and osteoarthritis is very commonly observed in several joints in the same cat.

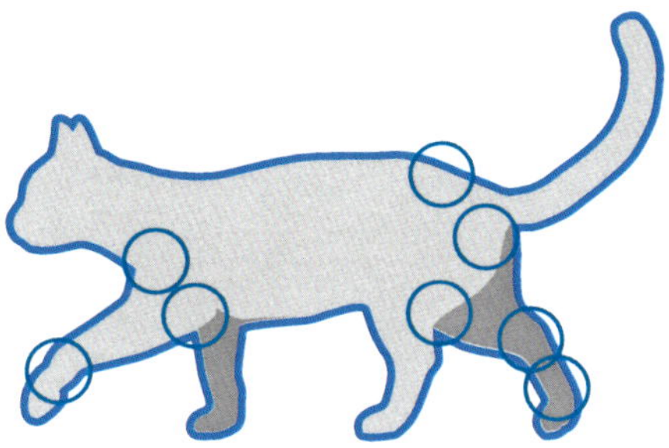

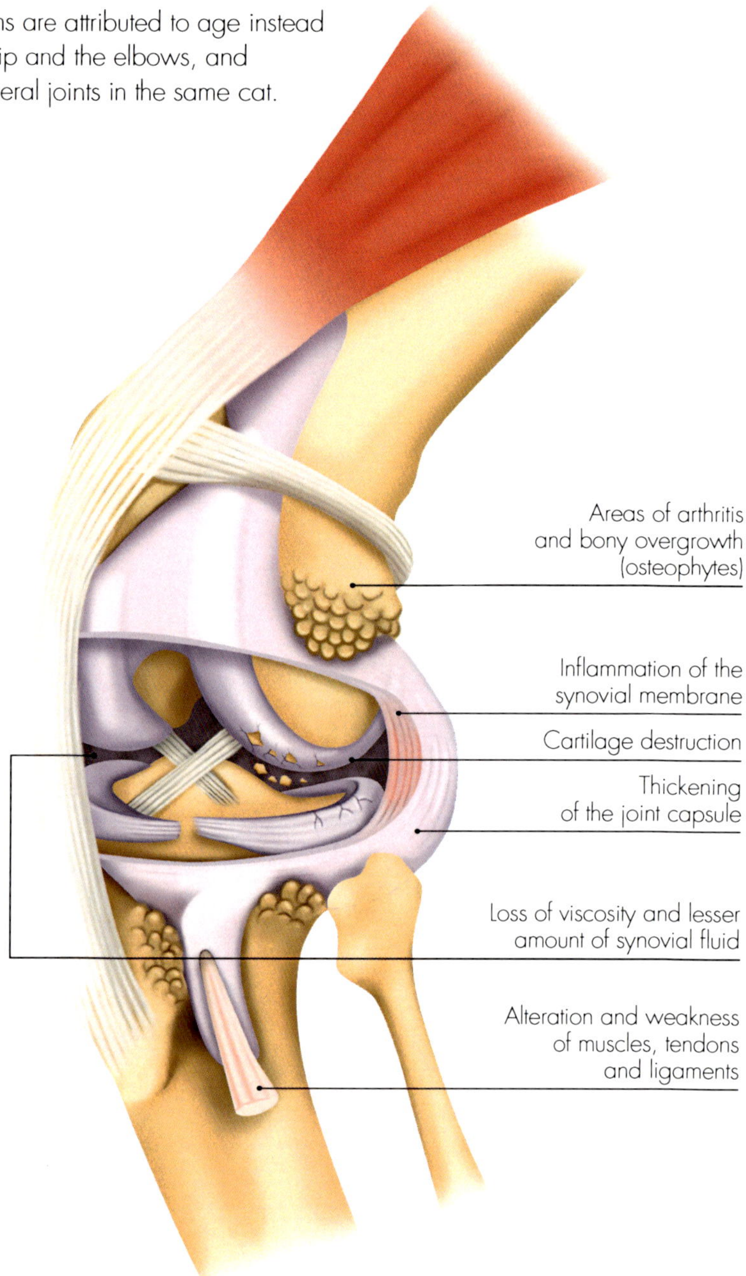

90 % of cats over 12 years of age show signs of joint degeneration.

What the owner sees

- The cat does not jump up to high surfaces, or uses intermediate steps to do so.
- It hesitates when trying to jump down.
- It does not play on a daily basis.
- It does not tolerate being brushed or being held in someone's arms, when it used to do so.
- More frequent meowing.
- Decreased grooming.

Medical treatment

Administration of analgesics over long periods of time.

Dietary treatment

Dietary modification, with diets rich in glycosaminoglycans and essential fatty acids.

Recommendations

- Prevention of obesity.
- Environmental modifications to facilitate mobility and access to the animal's favourite places.

MUSCULOSKELETAL SYSTEM

5 Hip dysplasia

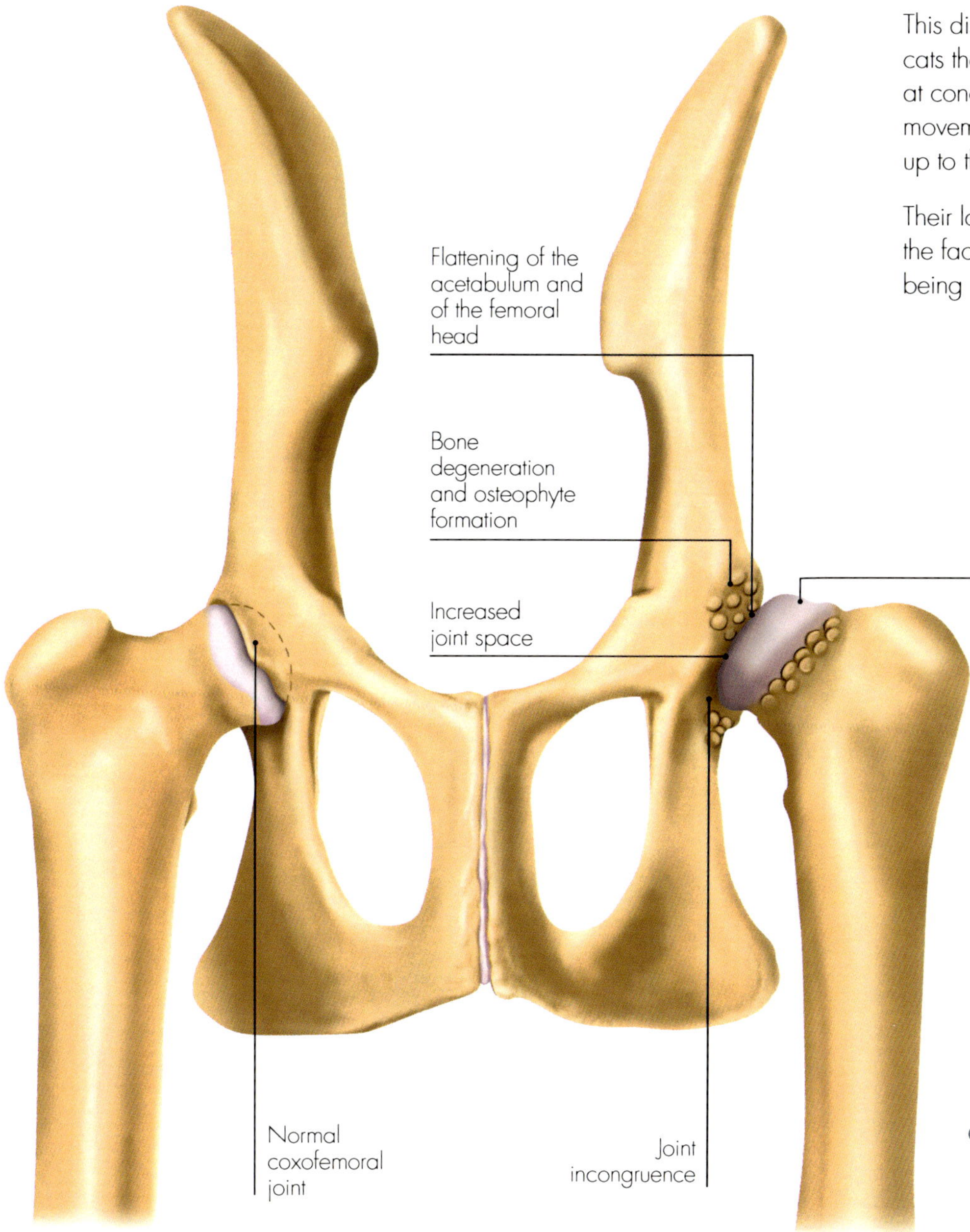

This disease is diagnosed less frequently in cats than in dogs because cats are very good at concealing their pain and avoid painful movements, using intermediate steps to jump up to their favourite places and playing less.

Their lack of activity is wrongly attributed to the fact that they are older, instead of to them being in pain.

It may occur in any cat, but the Maine Coon, Persian, Himalayan, Siamese, Bengal, Devon Rex and Abyssinian breeds are most commonly affected.

Clinical signs

In cats suffering from joint degeneration and osteoarthritis, we will observe:

- Stiffness of hind limbs when walking.
- Clumsier movements when jumping up to their favourite places or they may not reach high places in one jump.
- Lameness, although it is uncommon.
- Their daily play sessions are reduced.
- They may become more irritable when their hind limbs are touched.

MUSCULOSKELETAL SYSTEM

6 Sacrococcygeal luxation

Usual causes

- Abrupt pulling of the tail.
- Road traffic accidents.
- Dog bites.
- Other traumas (e.g. gunshots).

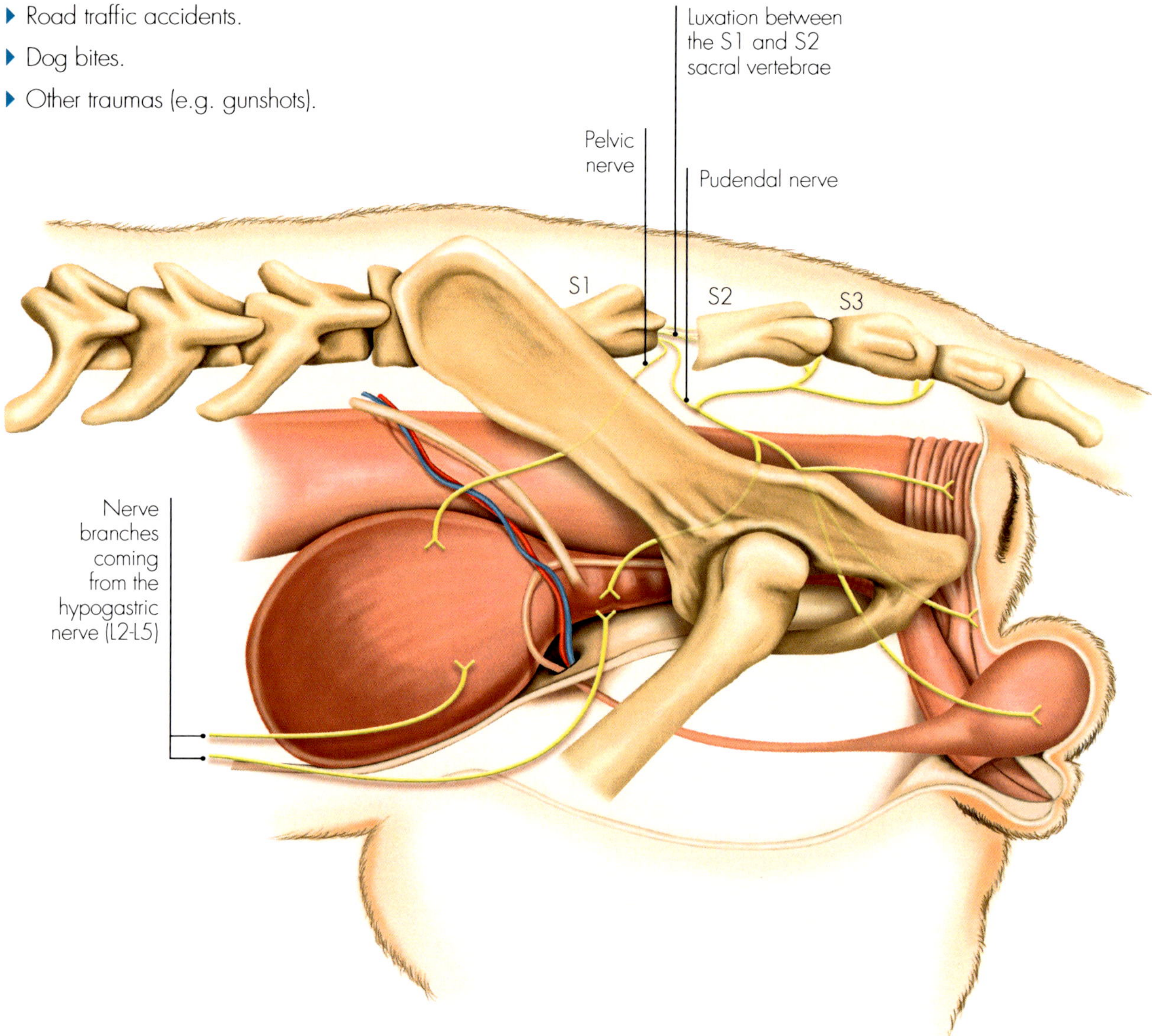

Clinical signs

- Problems of micturition (incontinence) and defecation and loss of perineal sensitivity due to:
  - Lesion of the pudendal nerve: sensory and motor innervation of the anal and urethral sphincters, and sensitivity of the perineum and genital organs.
  - Lesion of the pelvic nerves: innervation of the rectum, genitalia and detrusor muscle of the bladder. Urinary incontinence.
- Flaccidity or paralysis of the tail due to a lesion of the caudal nerves (sensory and motor innervations).
- Mild or moderate alterations in the hind limbs due to a secondary involvement of the sciatic nerve.

UROGENITAL SYSTEM

7 Chronic kidney disease (CKD)

It is one of the most common conditions in feline medicine. It affects animals at any age, but the probability of suffering from it doubles from 7-10 years of age. Cats do not show clinical signs until at least 70 % of the functional nephrons have been lost.

A precise diagnosis requires carrying out multiple tests such as blood tests, urinalysis, UPC ratio test, urine cultures, blood pressure measurement and diagnostic imaging techniques.

Normal kidney

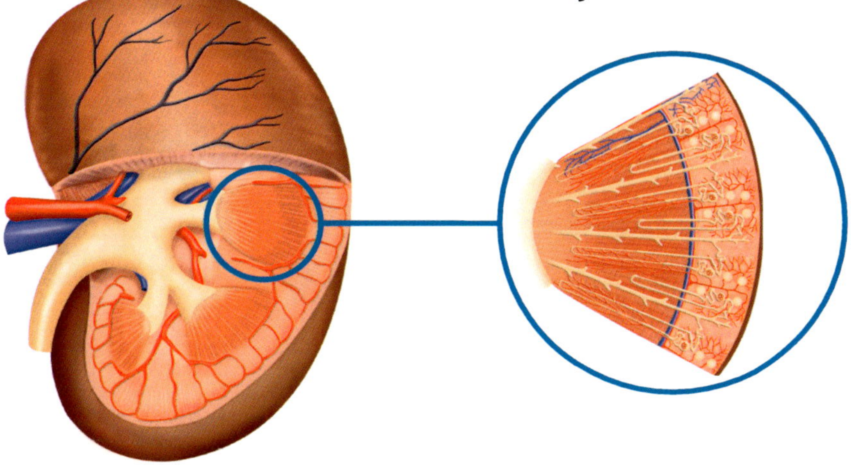

Kidney with CKD

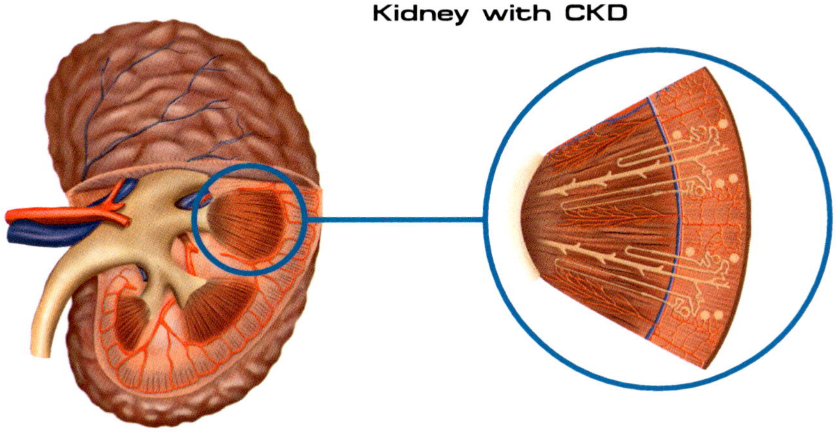

Progression of CKD

1. Kidney damage
2. Reduction of the number and function of nephrons
3. Progressive reduction of glomerular filtration
4. Increased levels of urea and creatinine and other products excreted by the kidneys
5. Onset of clinical signs: polyuria/polydipsia, progressive loss of weight, chronic vomiting, loss of appetite
6. If it progresses, it may lead to death

Causes of CKD

Congenital:

- Renal aplasia, dysplasia and hypoplasia.
- Renal amyloidosis.
- Feline polycystic kidney disease.

Acquired:

- Idiopathic tubulo-interstitial nephritis.
- Pyelonephritis.
- Glomerulonephritis.
- Acquired amyloidosis.
- Nephrotoxins.
- Hypercalcaemia.
- Hydronephrosis (chronic ureteral obstruction).
- Renal lymphoma.
- Progression of acute kidney disease.
- Feline infectious peritonitis.

UROGENITAL SYSTEM

8 Systemic hypertension (SH)

It is the sustained increase in arterial pressure (AP) above values considered as normal. Values of systolic AP > 140 mmHg obtained with an HDO device (high-definition oscillometry) and > 160 mmHg obtained with a Doppler ultrasound device are indicative of hypertension.

Blood pressure should be taken at least 10 minutes after the animal has entered the consultation room and 5 consecutive measurements must be made so as to calculate the mean value.

Causes

- Idiopathic or essential (the cause is unknown).
- Secondary to:
  - Kidney disease.
  - Hyperthyroidism.
  - After the treatment of hyperthyroidism (20 % of the cats treated).
  - Hyperaldosteronism.
  - Pheochromocytoma.
- White coat hypertension.

Consequences

- Hypertensive cats may be asymptomatic for months or years, until tissue damage is evident.
- Organs that suffer damage:
  - Heart.
  - Kidney.
  - Brain.
  - Eyes.

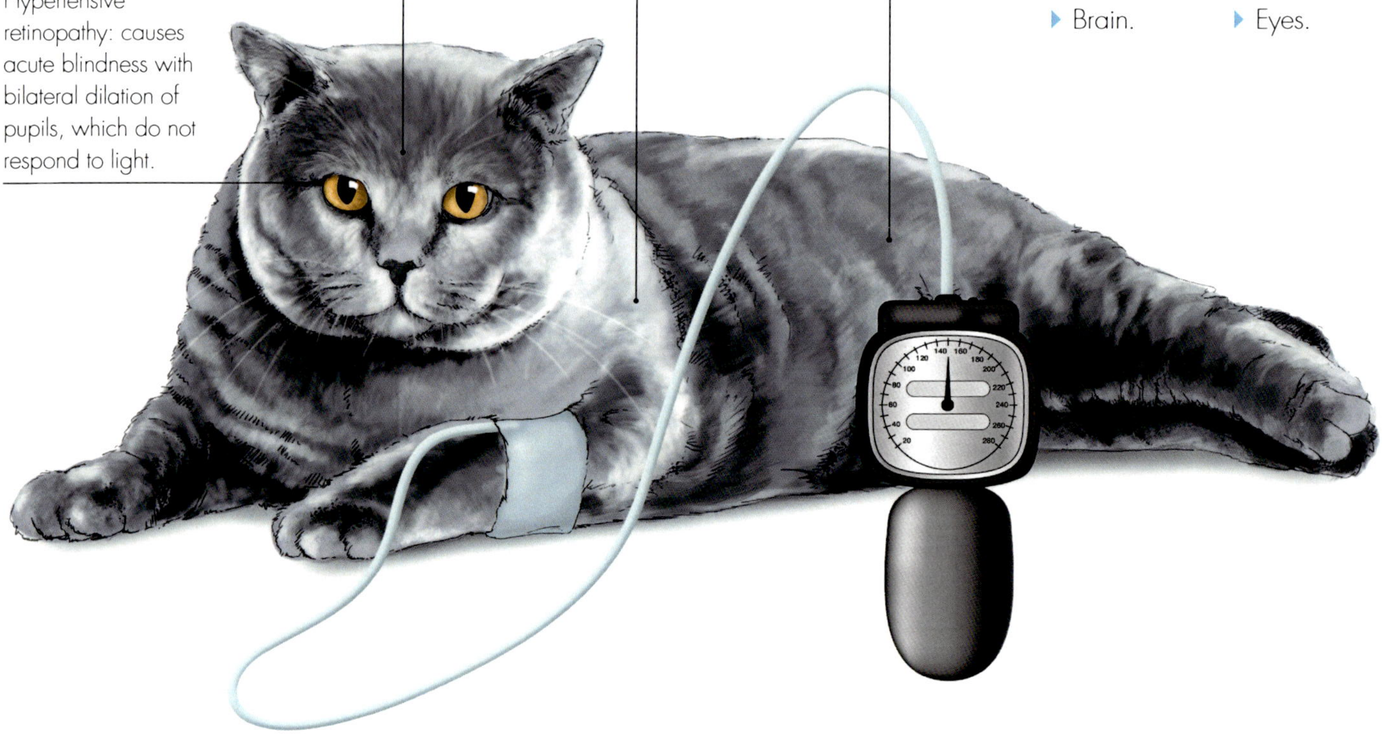
Hypertensive encephalopathy (disorientation, ataxia, convulsions, coma)
Cardiac hypertrophy (murmurs, cardiomegaly)
Contributes to progression of kidney disease
Hypertensive retinopathy: causes acute blindness with bilateral dilation of pupils, which do not respond to light.

UROGENITAL SYSTEM

9 Ureteral obstruction

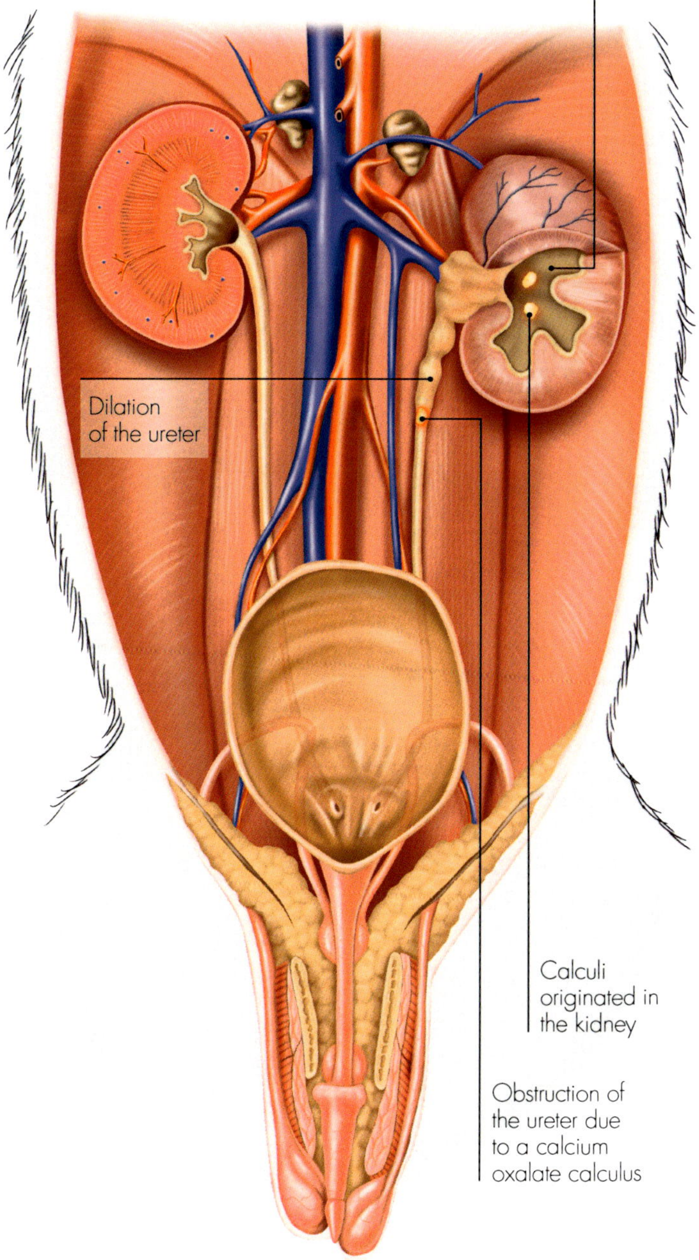

It is a frequent cause of chronic and acute kidney disease in cats of any age and sex. Bilateral ureteral obstruction is commonly observed.

Its diagnosis is made by means of abdominal radiographs and a high-definition ultrasound scan.

Causes

- Calcium oxalate calculi (most frequent cause).
- Plugs of inflammatory protein debris and crystals, secondary to pyelonephritis or to the previous migration of calculi.
- Plugs composed of more than 99 % blood with no associated crystals.
- Neoplasm in the bladder trigone (distal obstructions).
- Renal neoplasm (proximal obstructions).
- Post ureteral surgery obstructions.

Medical treatment

- Intravenous fluid therapy for azotaemia.
- Smooth muscle relaxants to facilitate passage of the calculus.
- Analgesics.

Surgical treatment

- Complicated due to the size of the ureter in cats.
- Obstruction in proximal ureter: ureterotomy or pyeloureterotomy.
- Obstruction in distal third of ureter: ureteroneocystotomy.

Dietary treatment

To avoid the formation of new calcium oxalate calculi.

UROGENITAL SYSTEM

10 Polycystic kidney disease (PKD)

This disease is hereditary and causes the formation of cysts in the kidneys. They are present from birth and, although they are initially very small, they grow over time and damage the kidney (kidney disease). They sometimes also affect the liver.

Breeds with a high risk: Persian, Exotic Shorthair, British Shorthair and crossbreeds of these breeds.

Breeds with a moderate risk: Birman, Burmilla, Devon Rex and Ragdoll.

Other breeds: very low risk.

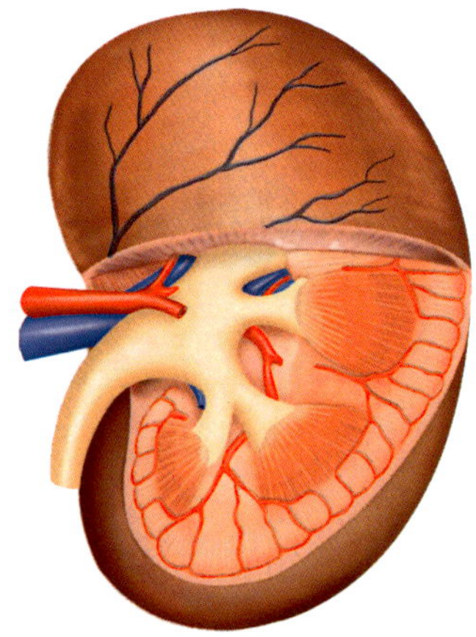

Normal kidney

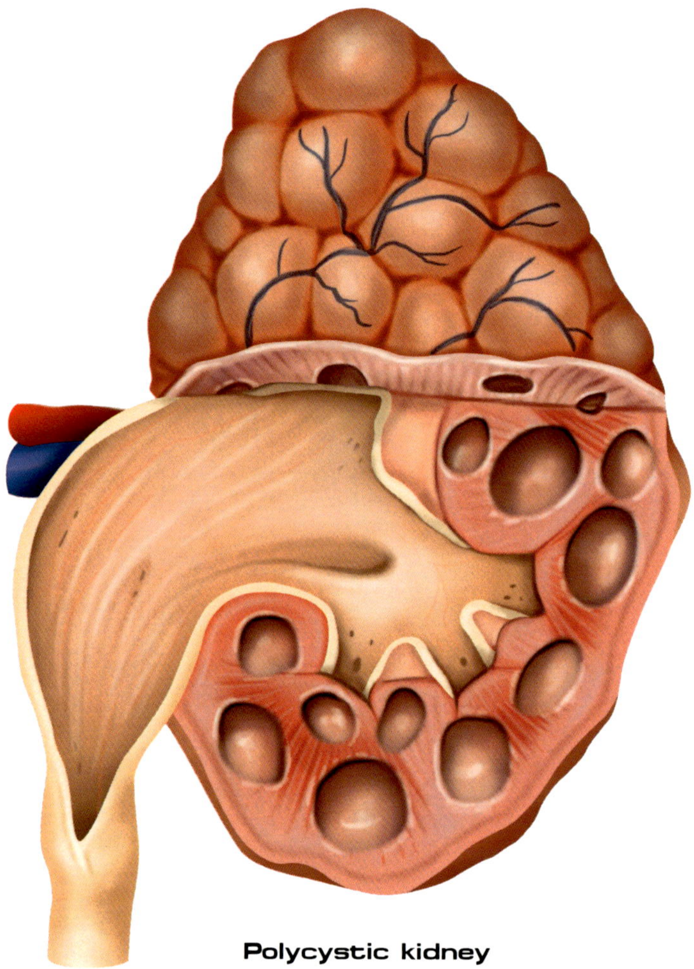

Polycystic kidney

Renal cysts

- Number: varies in each individual (from 20 to 200 cysts).
- Growth: it may be very fast (early death), or slow with symptoms of kidney disease from 8 years of age.
- Diagnosis:
  - Abdominal ultrasound.
  - Genetic testing with blood and saliva.

There are no treatments to prevent the progressive growth of cysts. Their growth speed is different in each cat and is determined by serial ultrasound studies.

Form of heredity

- It is transmitted by a single dominant autosomal gene; any cat with this gene will develop the disease.
- All the carriers of this gene are affected, even if they have few cysts.
- All the cats with the disease will transmit it to some of their offspring (approximately 50 %).

Medical treatment

Necessary in cats who develop kidney disease.

UROGENITAL SYSTEM

11 Feline lower urinary tract disease (FLUTD)

Obstructive and non-obstructive

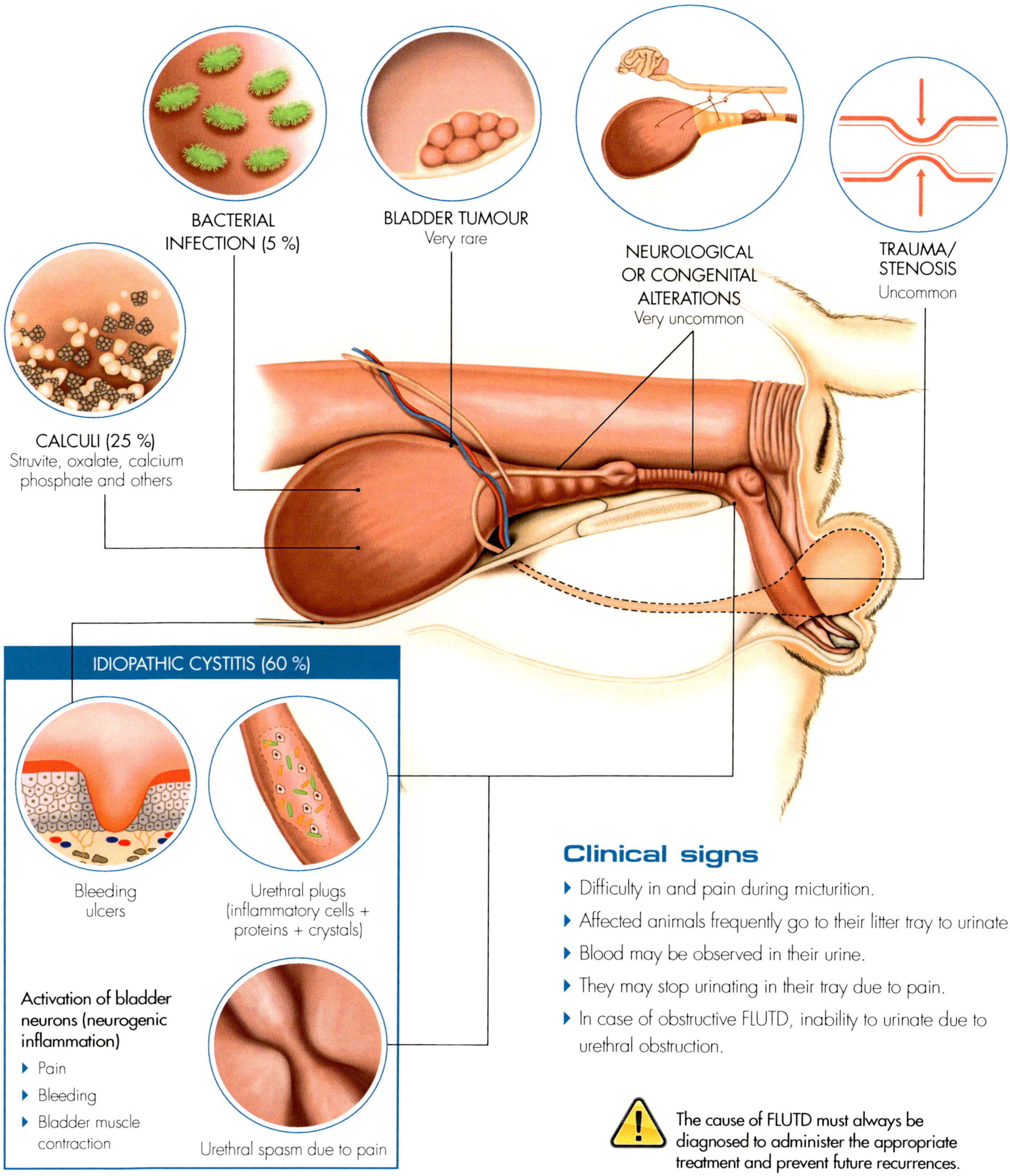

Clinical signs

- Difficulty in and pain during micturition.
- Affected animals frequently go to their litter tray to urinate.
- Blood may be observed in their urine.
- They may stop urinating in their tray due to pain.
- In case of obstructive FLUTD, inability to urinate due to urethral obstruction.

⚠ The cause of FLUTD must always be diagnosed to administer the appropriate treatment and prevent future recurrences.

UROGENITAL SYSTEM

12 Perineal urethrostomy

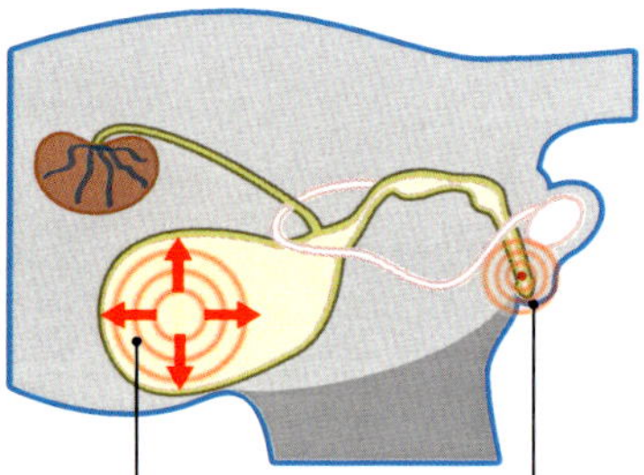

It involves creating an opening in the urethra and suturing it directly to the skin, in the perineal area below the anus, and removing the penis and testicles (if the cat is not already neutered).

Indications

- If the animal suffers from multiple obstructions (more than 3) despite treating FLUTD.
- Urethral obstruction impossible to resolve by means of catheterisation.
- Urethral stenosis.
- Severe penile injury.

Most complete urinary tract obstructions in cats are due to urethral plugs or to calculi.

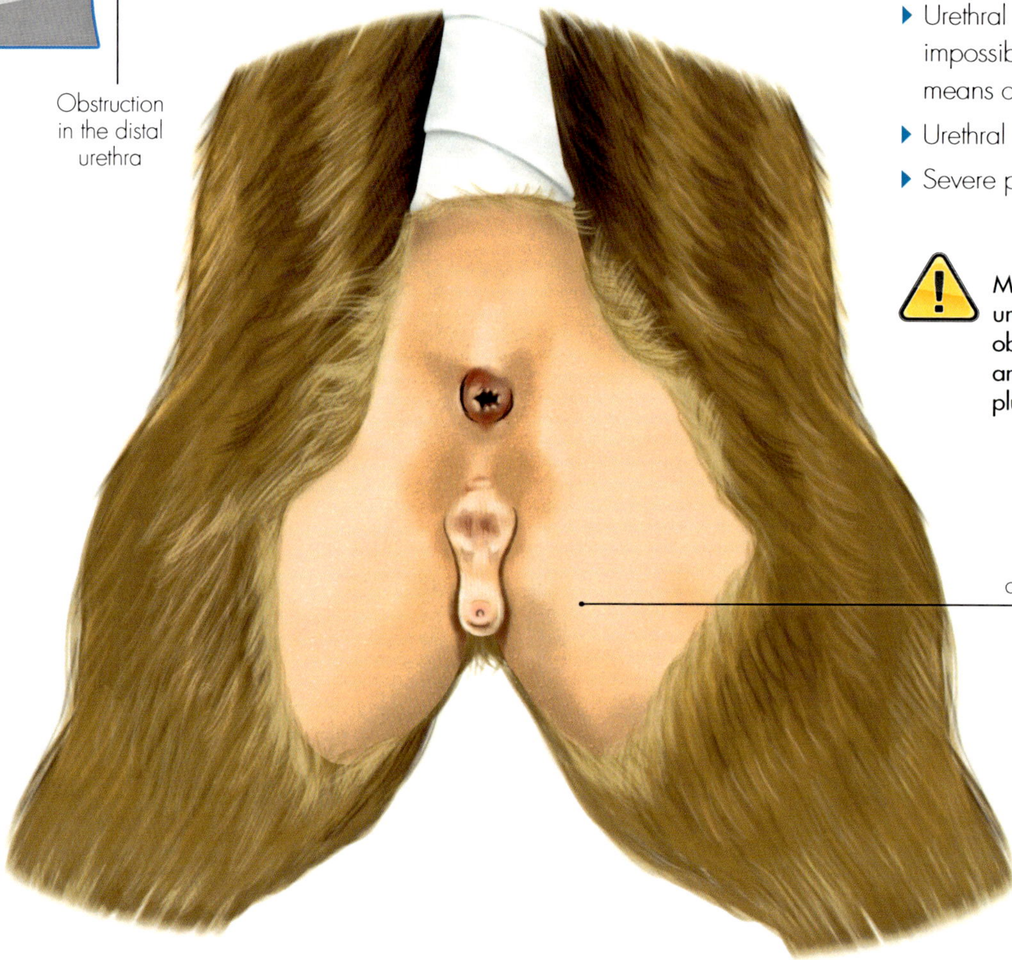

Surgical technique

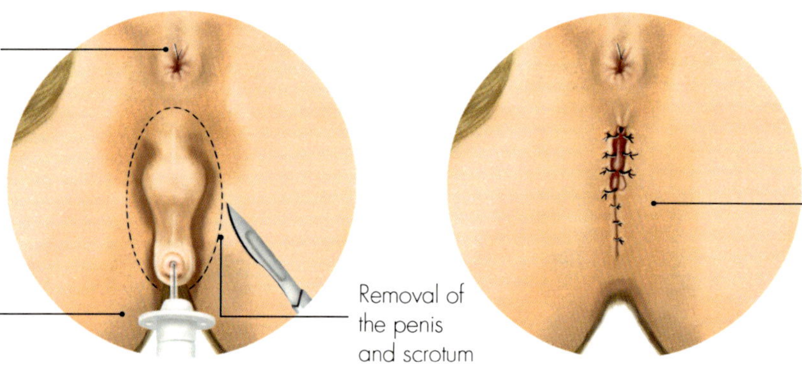

UROGENITAL SYSTEM

13 The oestrus cycle in female cats

Female cats are seasonally polyoestrous females, whose cycles are stimulated by an increasing photoperiod. They have regular cycles during the months of the year with longer periods of light (from February-March to October-November). Some females may also cycle all year round if they are exposed to artificial light.

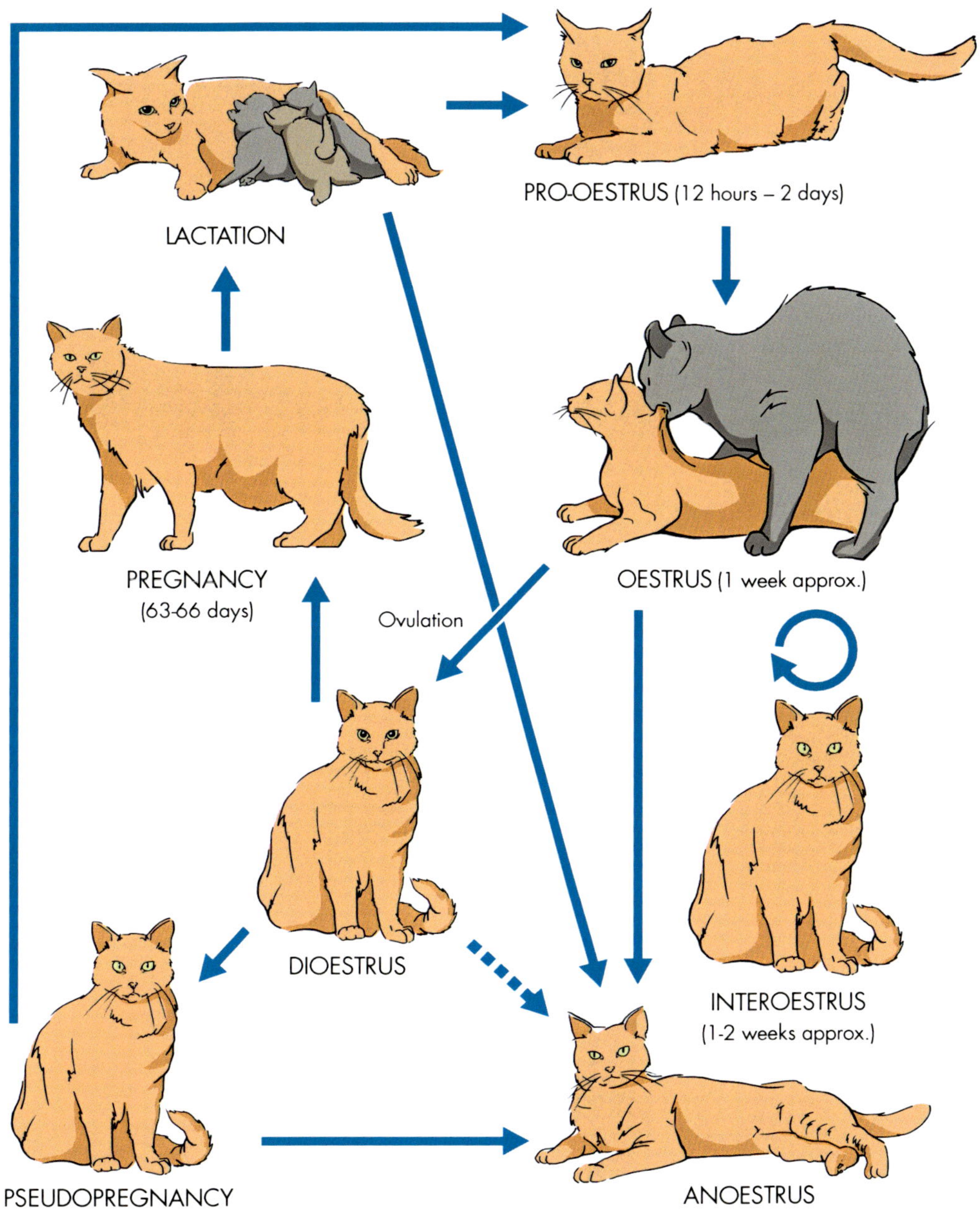

PRO-OESTRUS

- Males are attracted by non-receptive females.
- Mild vulvar oedema, with no bleeding (slight mucoid secretion).
- Sexual behaviour: purring, incessant meowing, lordosis behaviour, but does not allow mating.

OESTRUS

- Sexual behaviour similar to that of pro-oestrus, but the female allows mating.
- Ovulation induced by copulation. It may also be spontaneous.

INTEROESTRUS

- Appears when ovulation does not occur.
- Phase of inactivity between two consecutive heat cycles.

DIOESTRUS

- If ovulation takes place, the corpus luteum is formed (progesterone).
- Two situations may occur:
  - Pseudopregnancy: the cat ovulates, but there is no fertilisation.
  - Pregnancy: the cat ovulates and there is fertilisation.

ANOESTRUS

- Period with no sexual activity (absence of oestrus cycles).
- Between October-November and January-February (shorter periods of light). It may not appear under artificial light conditions.

⚠ They reach puberty between 6-8 months of age, although it may vary (4-12 months) depending on the weight, breed, etc.

⚠ The use of hormonal treatments to inhibit heat cycles should be avoided during the pro-oestrus and oestrus phases.
The moment of choice is usually the anoestrus phase.

UROGENITAL SYSTEM

14 Neutering

in males and females

Ovariohysterectomy — Female

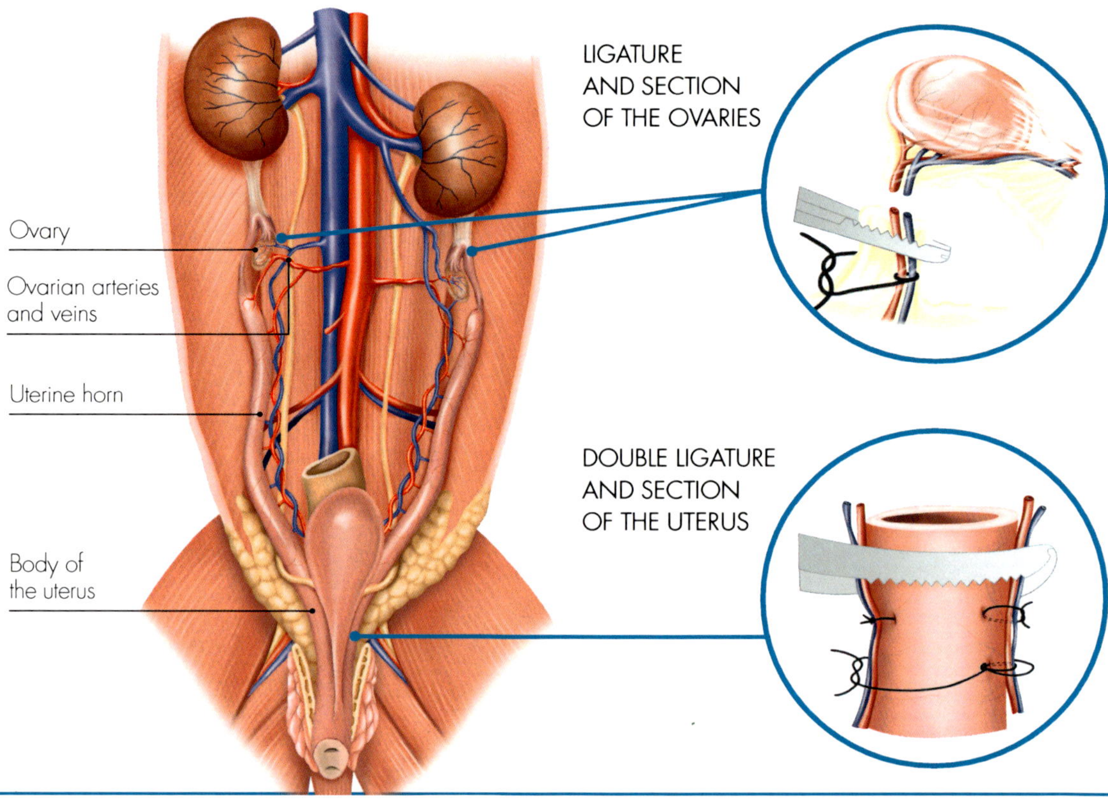

Orchiectomy — Male

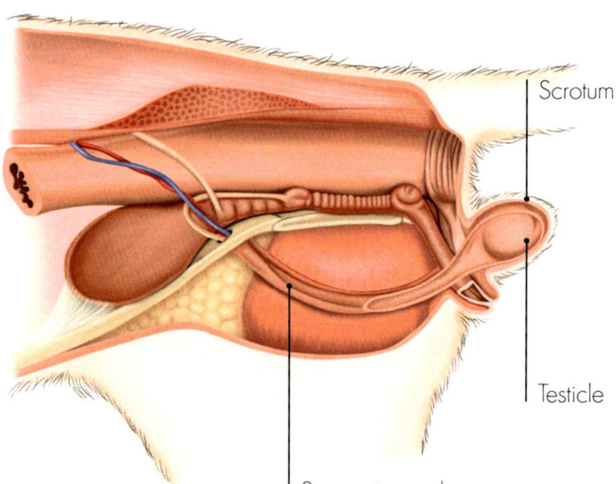

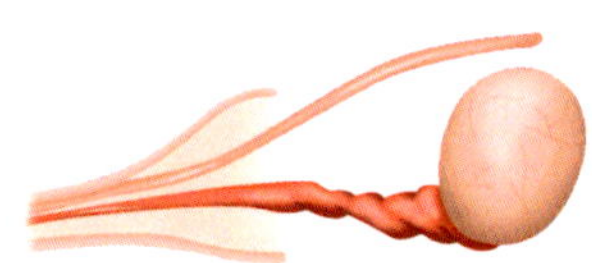

The vas deferens is separated from the testicle and blood vessels.

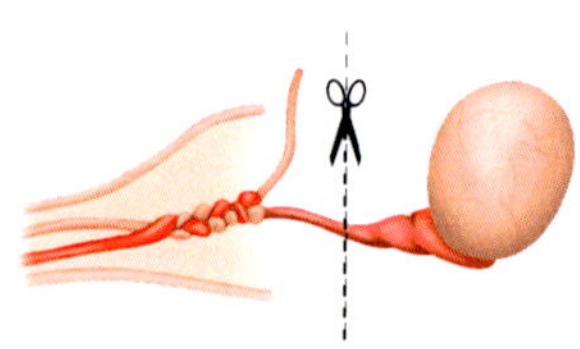

The vas deferens is tied around the blood vessels and the testicle is then sectioned. It is also possible to use sutures to ligate the vessels and duct.

UROGENITAL SYSTEM

15 Pyometra

Infection of the uterus

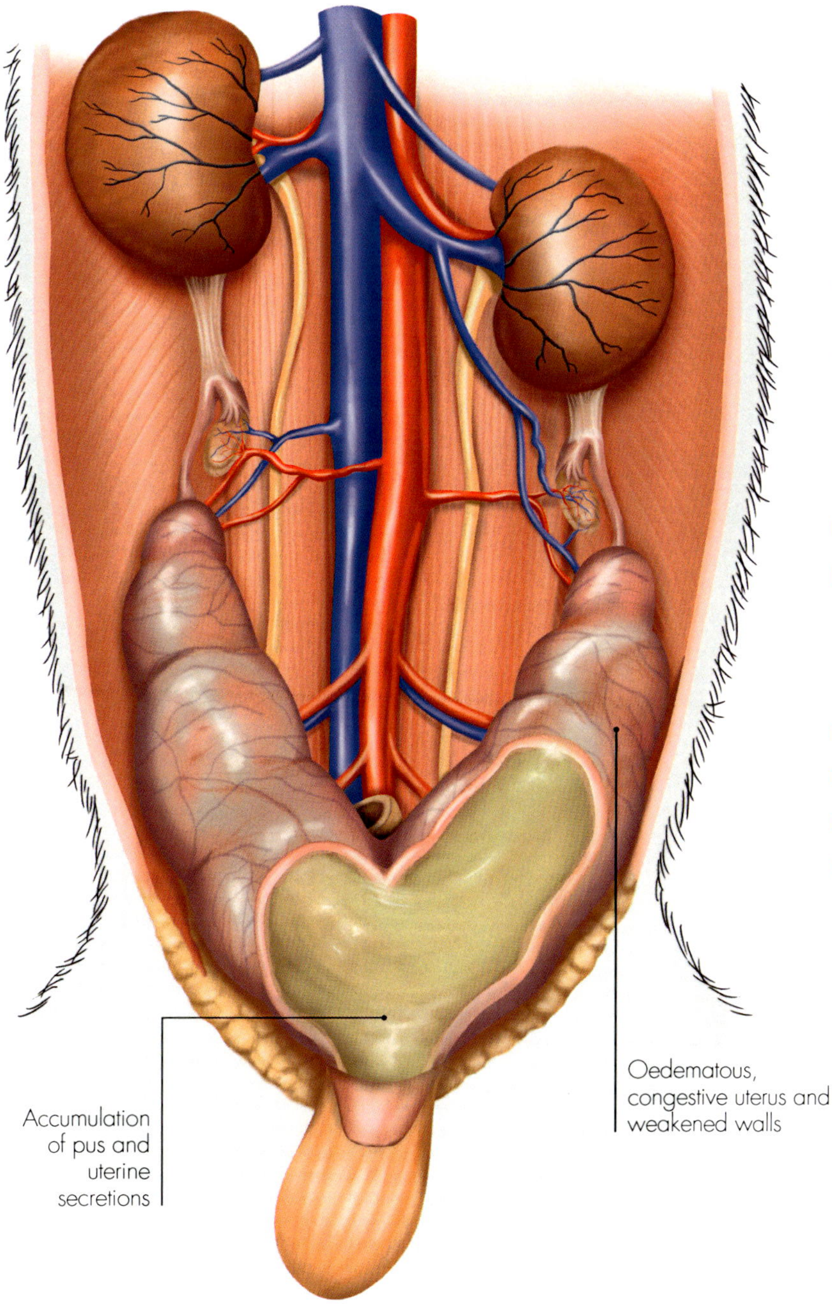

Infectious disease caused by bacteria and characterised by the presence of pus within the uterine cavity. It occurs in female cats of any age, regardless of whether they have already had kittens. The use of progestogens to inhibit oestrus is a risk factor.

Its diagnosis requires the use of abdominal radiography and ultrasonography.

Clinical signs

- Serous-bloody or mucopurulent vaginal discharge. If it is a closed-cervix pyometra, no secretions will be observed.
- Lethargy.
- Loss of weight.
- Polyuria and polydipsia.
- Fever is not common.

Medical treatment

- Fluid therapy.
- Antibiotics.
- Hormones until its resolution.

Surgical treatment

Treatment of choice (ovariohysterectomy), especially if it is not a breeding female and if signs of severe infection such as peritonitis are observed.

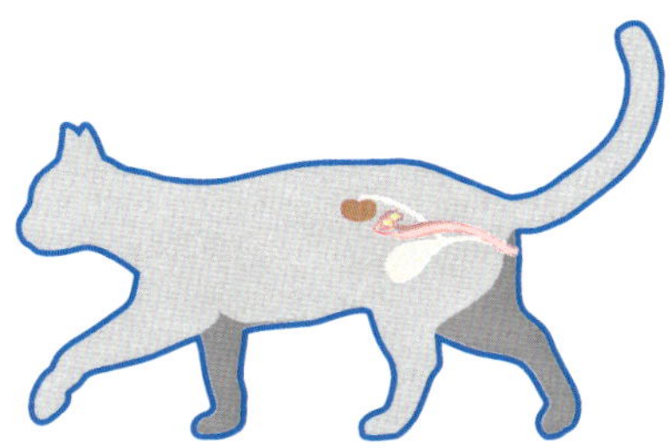

UROGENITAL SYSTEM

16 Mammary tumours

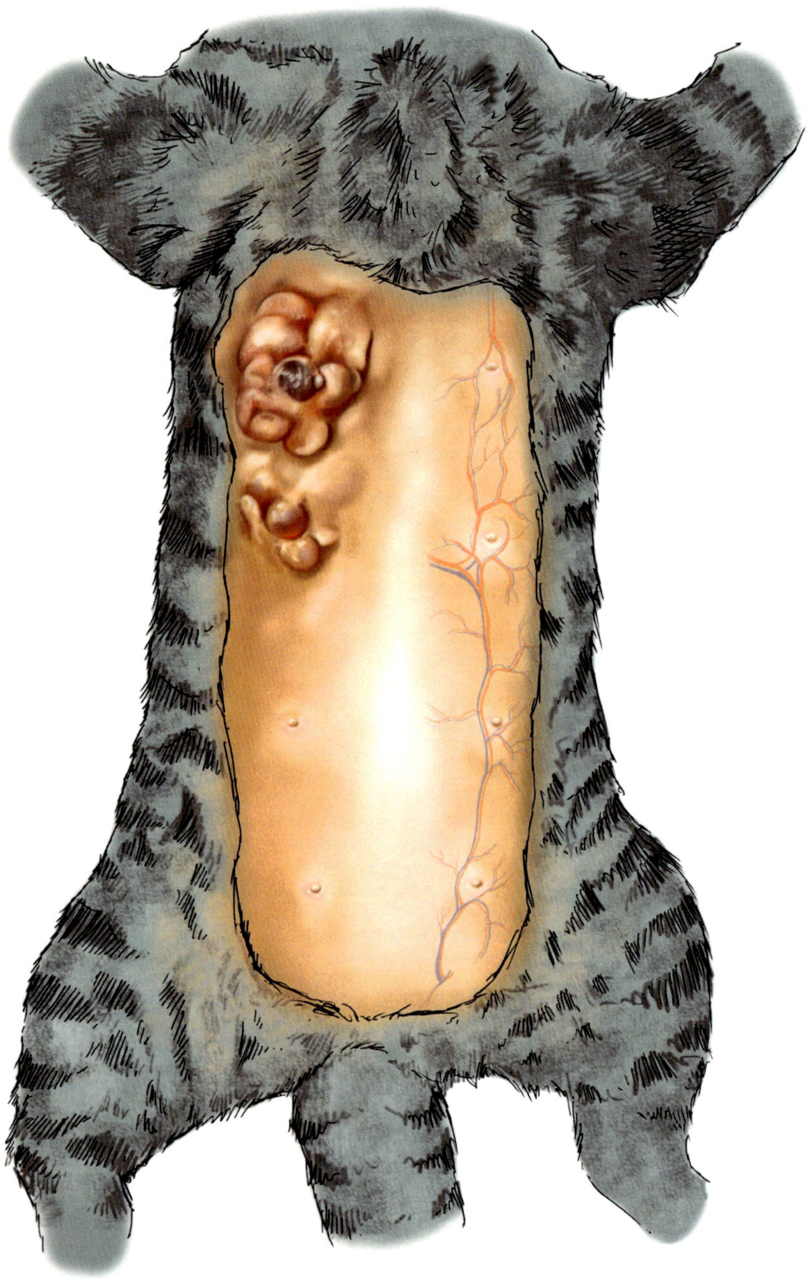

In cats, 80-96 % of mammary tumours are malignant, the most frequent ones being tubular and papillary adenocarcinomas. Barely 10 % of cases are adenomas. Only 1-2 % of mammary tumours occur in males. The average age of presentation is 11 years, although it may affect younger female cats. The diagnosis of mammary tumours requires a biopsy, and thoracic radiography and abdominal ultrasonography to rule out the presence of metastases.

The risk of carcinoma is 6-7 times lower in females neutered before 6 months of age.

Clinical signs

Size is the most important factor:

- One or several firm, lobulated masses, which are occasionally ulcerated if they are large.
- Frequent local glandular involvement.
- Metastases in the lung and organs such as the liver and lymph nodes, very common in nodules > 3 cm.

The use of progestogens to control oestrus cycles increases the risk of developing mammary tumours or adenomatous hyperplasia.

Surgical treatment

Radical surgery, removing the entire mammary chain, reduces the risk of recurrence (relapse).

Medical treatment

Chemotherapy may increase the interval between relapses as well as life expectancy.

Prognosis

Size is the most important factor:

- Female cats with tumours < 2 cm may live up to 3 years after the surgery.
- Cats with tumours < 3 cm live for about 4-6 months.

CARDIORESPIRATORY SYSTEM

17 Cardiorespiratory system

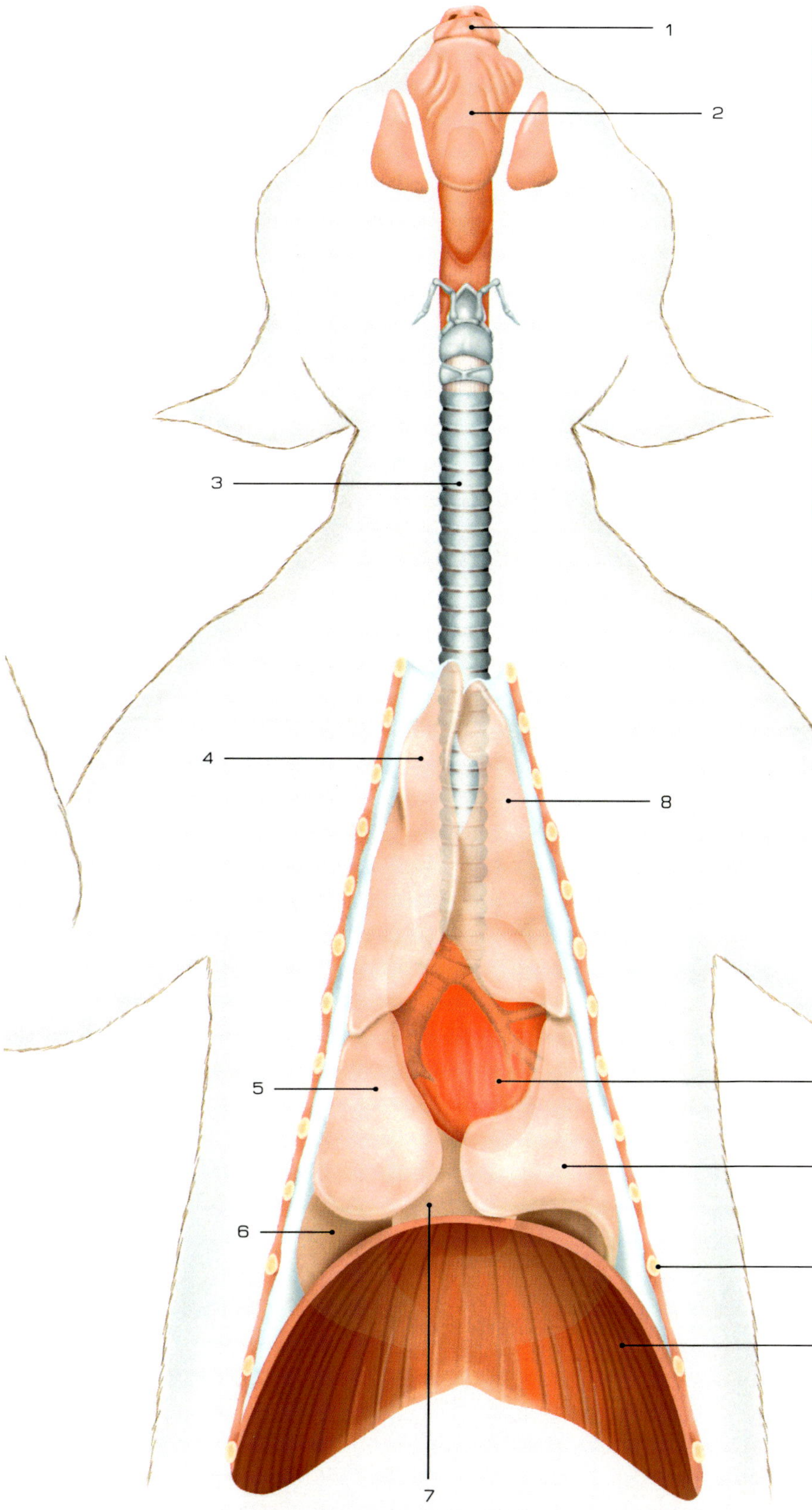

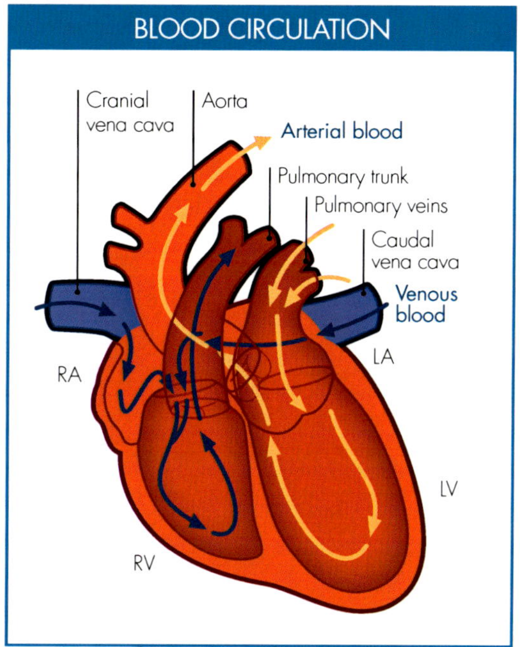

1. Nose
2. Nasal cavity
3. Trachea
4. Right lung, cranial lobe
5. Right lung, middle lobe
6. Right lung, caudal lobe
7. Right lung, accessory lobe
8. Left lung, cranial lobe
9. Left lung, caudal lobe
10. Heart
11. Ribs
12. Diaphragm

CARDIORESPIRATORY SYSTEM

18 Brachycephaly in cats

The brachycephalic conformation of the skull in Persian and Himalayan cats causes obstruction of the upper airways, disorders of the tear drainage system and alters the structure of the teeth. The more brachycephalic their skull is, the more severe these signs will be.

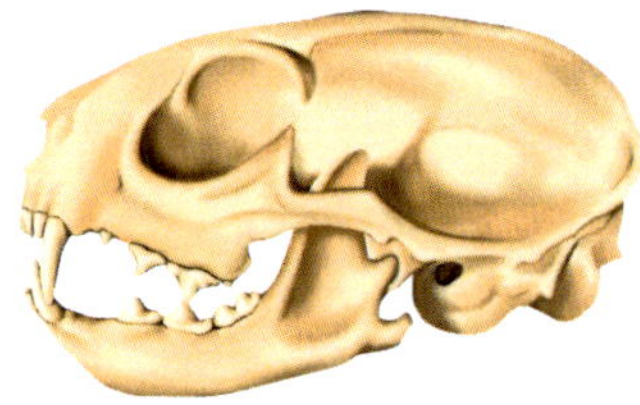

Normal skull

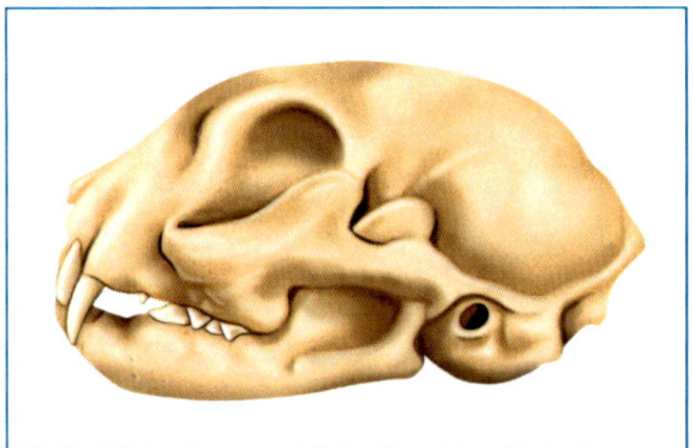

Grade I: mild

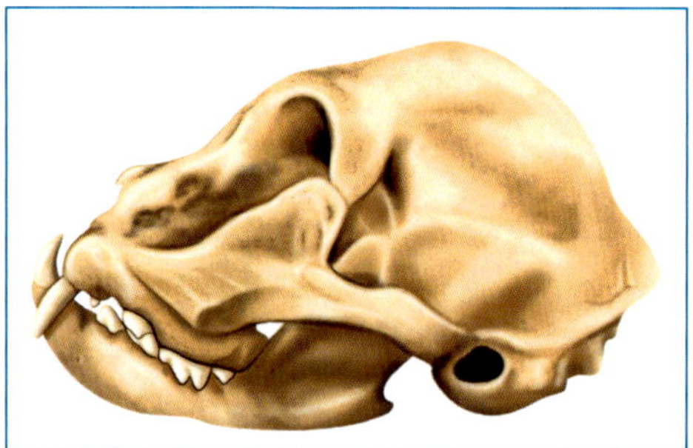

Grade II: moderate

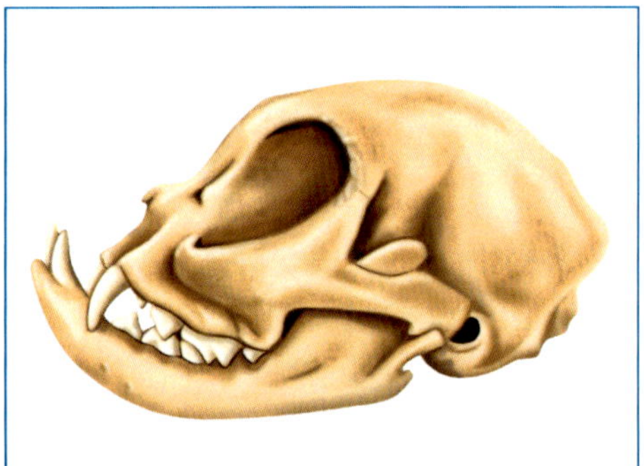

Grade III: intense

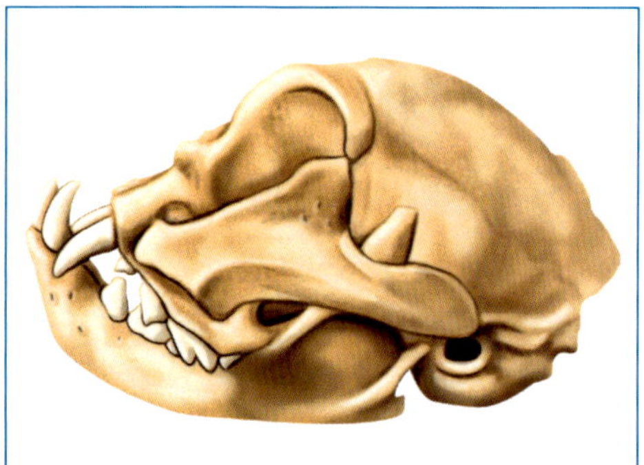

Grade IV: severe

Clinical signs

The higher the degree of brachycephaly, the more severe the signs will be:

- Alteration of the tear duct: constant tearing and secondary dermatitis.
- Greater exposure of the eyes: keratitis and corneal sequestra.
- Incorrect teeth alignment: difficulties in chewing and more frequent periodontal disease.
- Obstruction of the upper airways due to:
  - Stenotic nares.
  - Narrow nasal cavity.
  - Elongated soft palate.

Medical treatment

- In case of dermatitis of skinfolds due to epiphora.
- In case of keratitis.

Surgical treatment

- Surgical correction of stenotic nares and elongated soft palate.
- Removal of the teeth that prevent proper chewing.

Recommendations

The international veterinary community recommends the prohibition to breed cats with extreme brachycephaly due to the negative consequences on their health and life expectancy.

CARDIORESPIRATORY SYSTEM

19 Nasopharyngeal polyps

They are benign masses that may be located in the nasopharynx, Eustachian tube, tympanic cavity, or in the three locations at the same time. The most frequent presentation is in young cats of up to 5 years of age, although they may appear at any age.

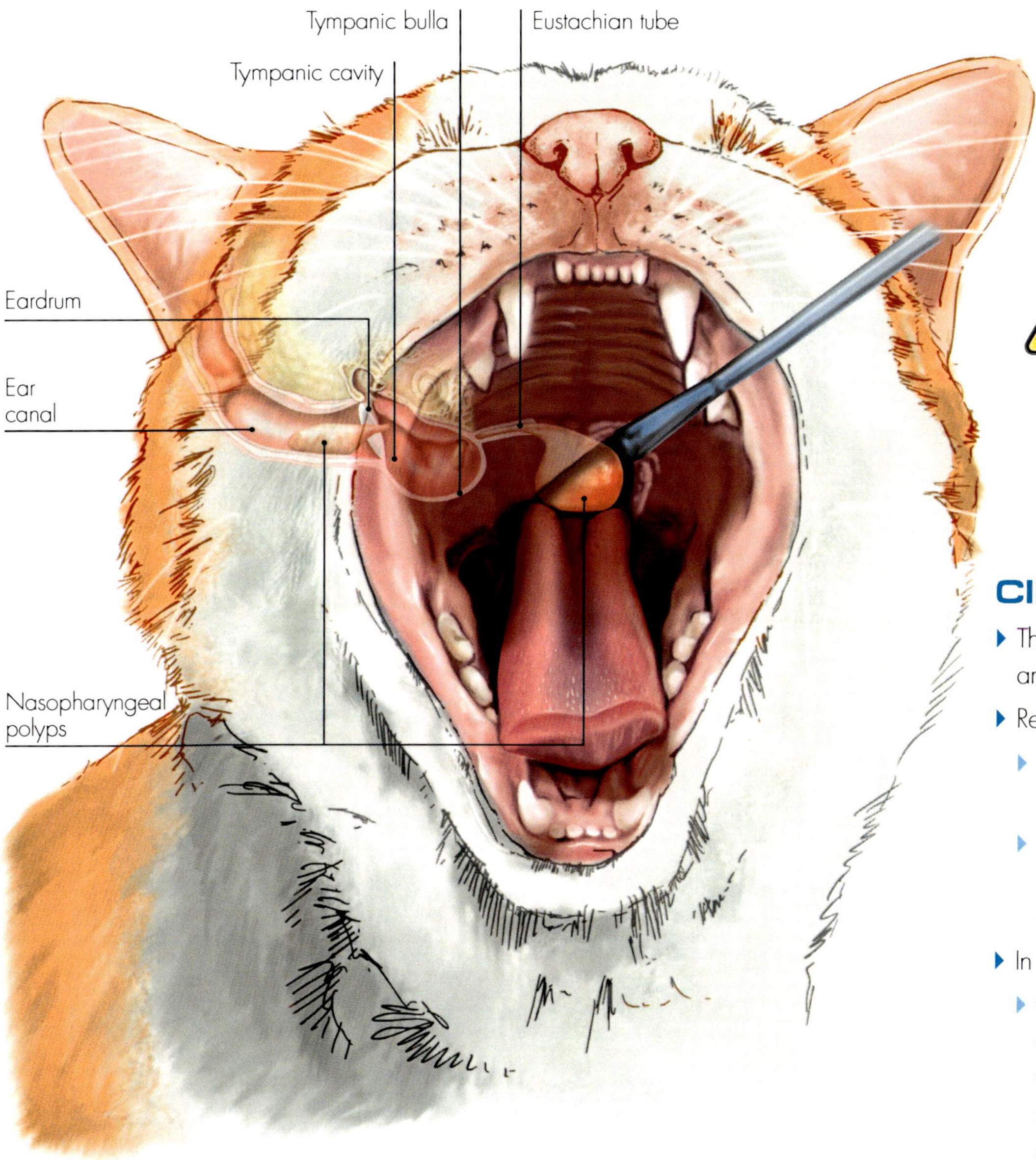

⚠ They are secondary to inflammatory or infectious processes of the respiratory tract or middle ear.

Clinical signs

- They are chronic and progressive, and affect the airways or inner ear.
- Respiratory:
  - Rhinitis and sinusitis with chronic nasal secretion and sneezing.
  - Dysphagia, cyanosis and syncope in case of obstruction of the airways.
- In the inner ear:
  - Otitis externa, media or interna, depending on their extension, with ear secretion, head tilt, nystagmus, vestibular ataxia and Horner's syndrome.

Medical treatment

- Gentle pulling from the nasopharynx or from the ear canal with the help of forceps.
- If the radiograph of the tympanic bullae shows opacity due to the presence of material, a previous antibiotic treatment may be given over a 4-week period before performing an osteotomy.

Surgical treatment

If the radiograph or CAT scan shows signs of involvement of the bone of the tympanic bullae: osteotomy.

CARDIORESPIRATORY SYSTEM

20 Dilated cardiomyopathy

The anomalous dilation of the cardiac muscle may be originated by a deficiency in taurine (cats fed with dog food), be idiopathic (in most cases), or appear as the end stage of a non-diagnosed valvular disease or of a myocardial ischaemic disease.

Breed predisposition: Siamese, Burmese and Abyssinian.

Normal heart

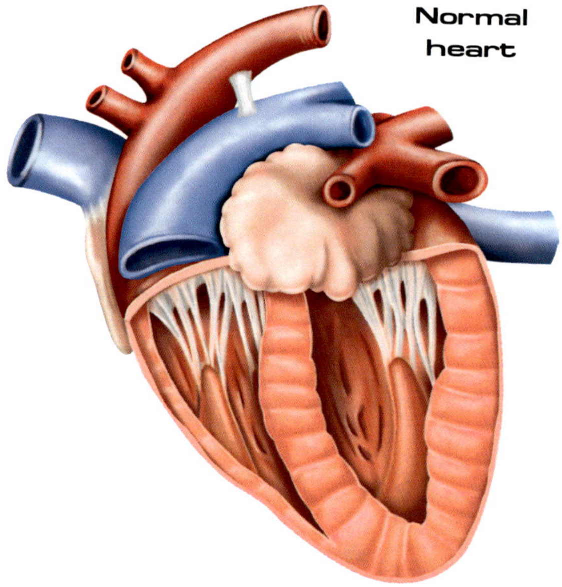

Dilated heart

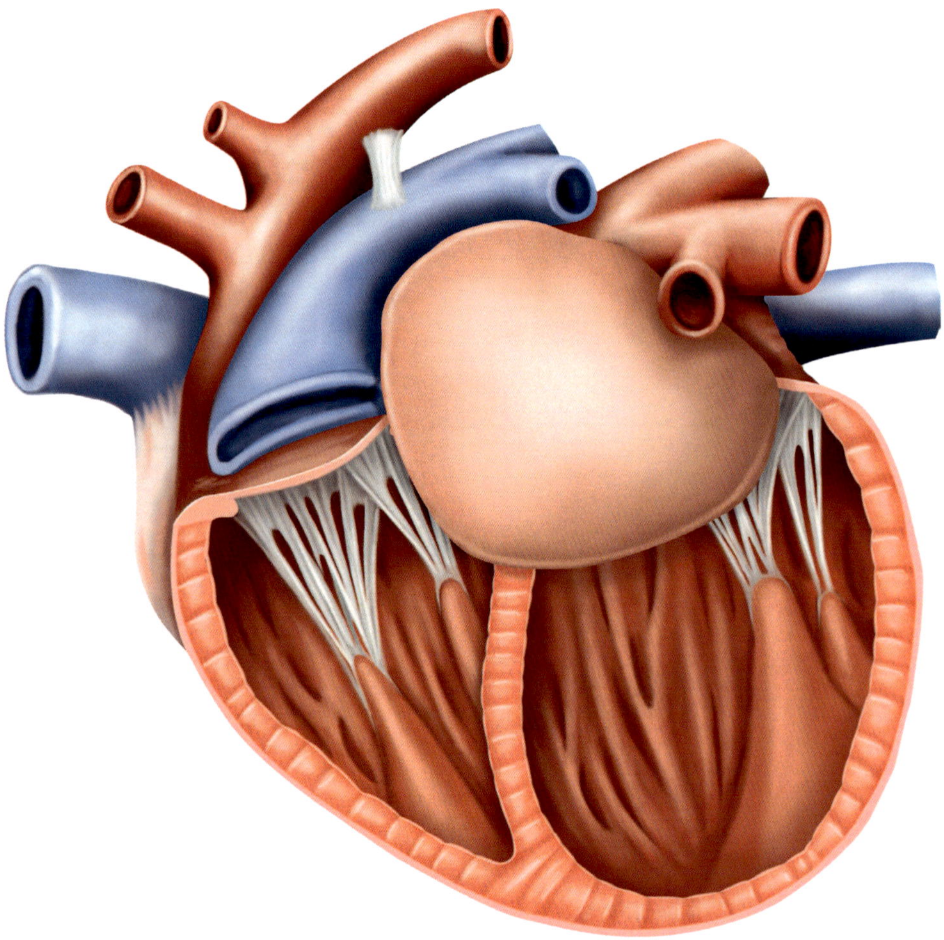

Clinical signs

- Murmur (approx. 60 % of cats with cardiomyopathy).
- Galloping rhythm.
- Limb paralysis caused by aortic thromboembolism (7 % of cats).
- Acute respiratory distress due to pulmonary oedema and/or pleural effusion.
- Progressive weight loss and weakness.

The animal may not show any signs until the disease is very advanced, which is why an early diagnosis by means of echocardiography is essential.

Medical treatment

Taurine levels should always be measured since its administration may correct the disease.

Taurine

- Essential amino acid for the normal functioning of the cardiac muscle, sight and reproduction, among other functions.
- Cats cannot synthesise it in a sufficient amount and must therefore obtain it from their diet.
- Its deficiency may cause: blindness, dilated cardiomyopathy, insufficient growth and poor reproductive results.

CARDIORESPIRATORY SYSTEM

21 Hypertrophic cardiomyopathy

Cardiomyopathy is more frequent in cats. It may be primary or secondary to hyperthyroidism, hypertension, obstruction of the outflow tract, acromegaly or myocardial neoplasia, and these conditions must therefore be ruled out. There may not be any clinical signs until it is very advanced, which is why an early diagnosis by means of echocardiography is essential.

Normal heart

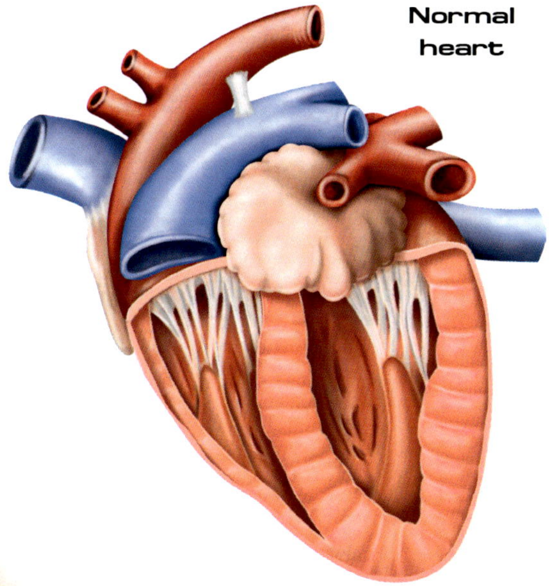

Hypertrophic heart

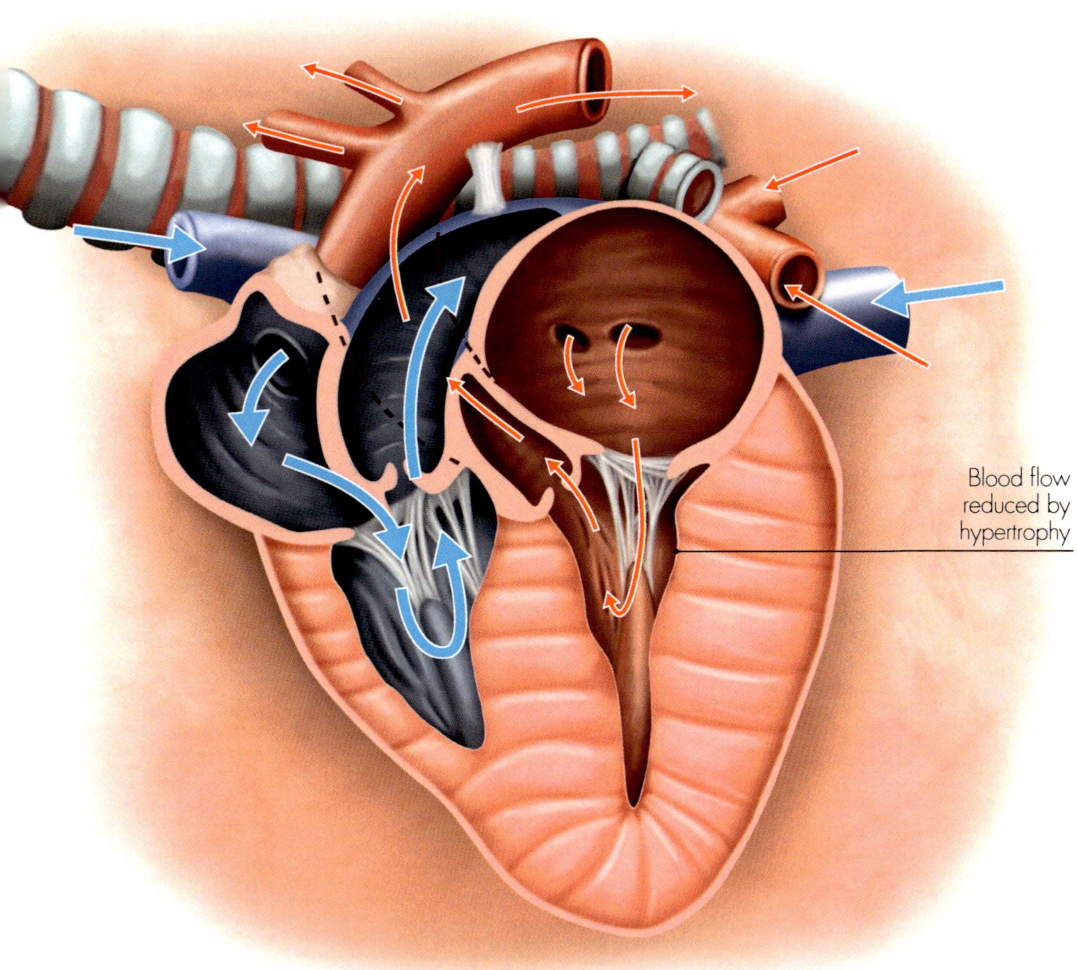

It affects almost all the breeds, although there is a genetic predisposition in the Maine Coon, Ragdoll, Norwegian Forest and British Shorthair.

The left ventricle cannot be filled properly due to the hypertrophy of its wall (diastolic dysfunction).

Medical treatment

Each stage requires a different type of treatment and no specific treatment is currently recommended at very early stages.

Clinical signs

- Murmur (approx. 60 % of cats with cardiomyopathy).
- Galloping rhythm.
- Limb paralysis caused by aortic thromboembolism (7 % of cats).
- Acute respiratory distress due to pulmonary oedema and/or pleural effusion.

CARDIORESPIRATORY SYSTEM

22 Arterial thromboembolism

Frequent complication associated with all types of cardiomyopathy in cats. Other causes of thromboembolism are: arterial thrombosis due to a vascular lesion, infection or tumours (pulmonary carcinomas).

On rare occasions, the forelimbs, cerebral, renal or mesenteric arteries may be affected.

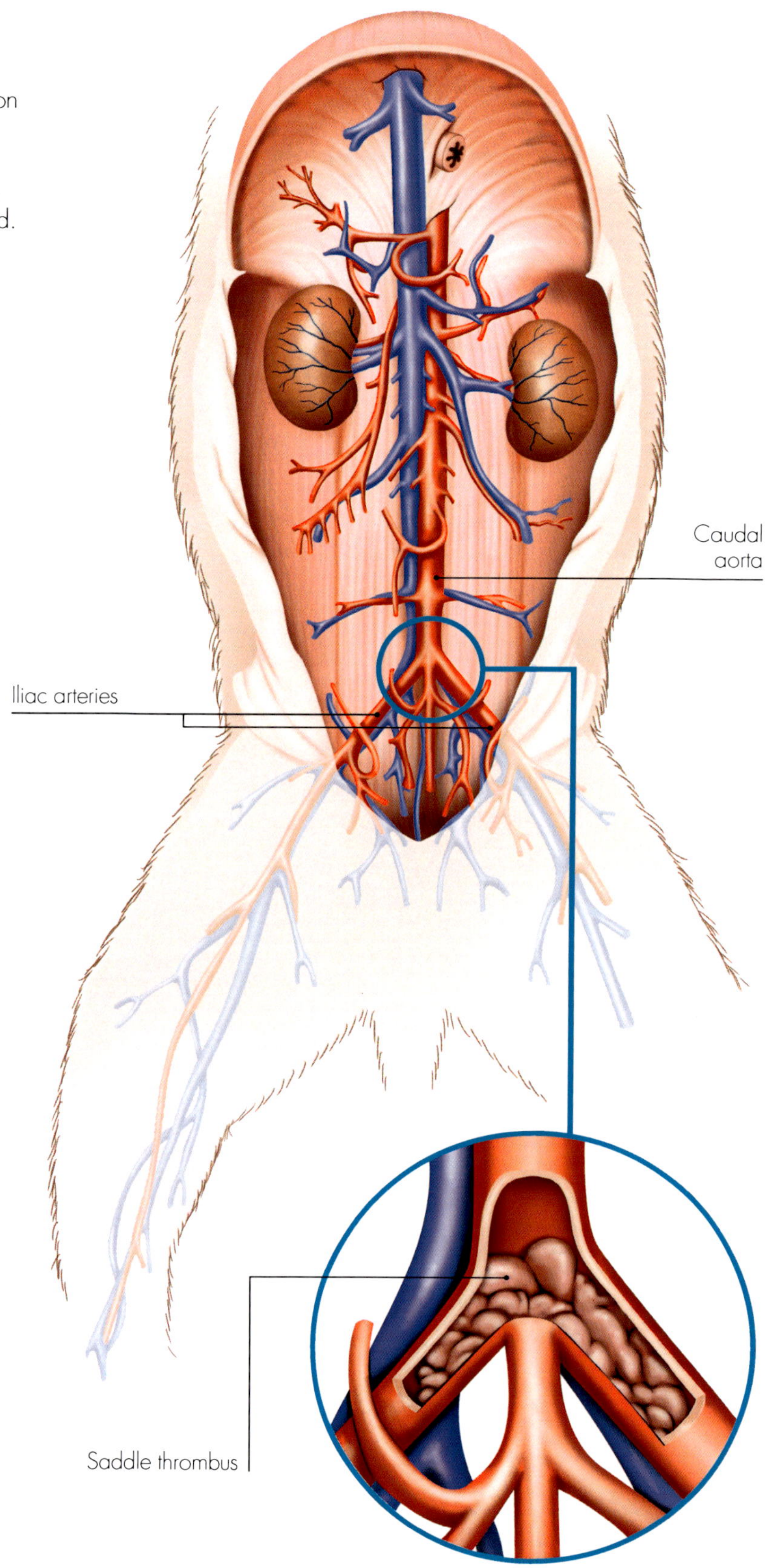

Clinical signs

- Acute excruciating pain.
- Paralysis or paresis of the affected limbs.
- The affected limbs do not have a pulse, are pale and cold.
- Some cats will also have signs of congestive heart failure.

Prognosis

- Poor, since mortality is high.
- Cats with only one affected limb usually have a better prognosis.

Most thrombi are located at the bifurcation of the aorta, which causes paralysis of one or two hind limbs.

CARDIORESPIRATORY SYSTEM

23 Feline asthma

Feline asthma (chronic allergic bronchitis) is the most frequent bronchopulmonary disease in cats. It occurs due to hypersensitivity reactions to inhaled allergens (dust, pollen, mites) or other factors (changes of temperature, drugs, exercise, infections, etc.), which cause chronic inflammation of the lower airways with an increase in the production of mucus and bronchoconstriction.

Its diagnosis requires thoracic radiographs and a bronchoalveolar lavage to rule out pulmonary infections and parasites.

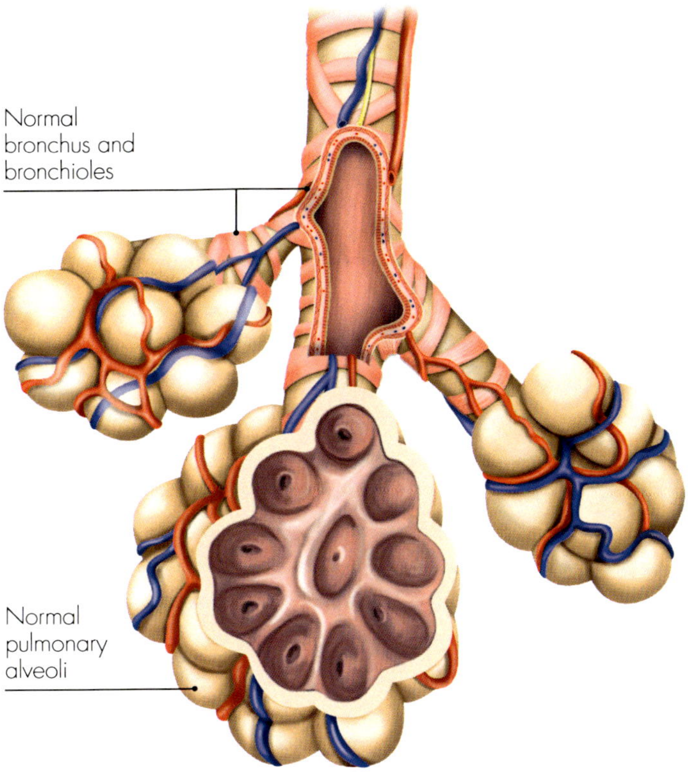

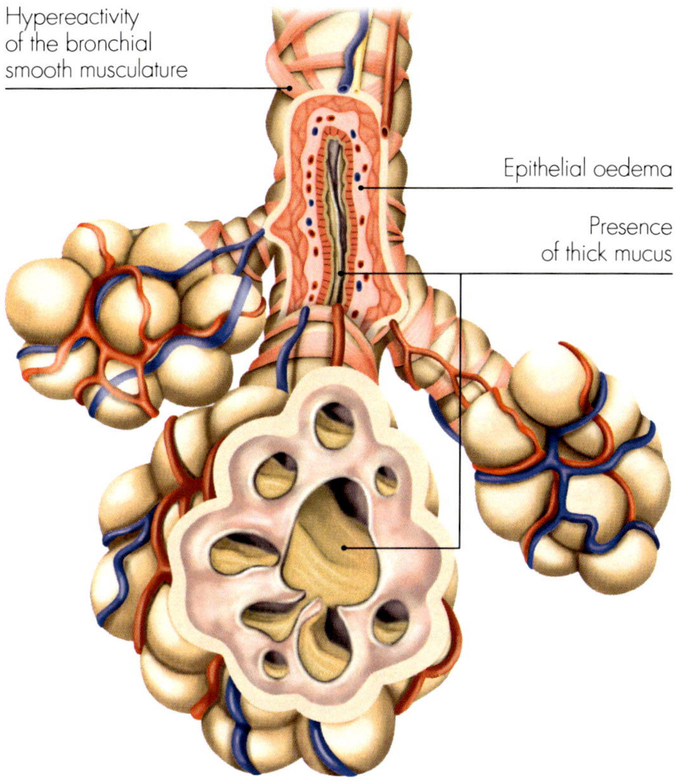

Clinical signs

- Chronic or intermittent cough with a variable intensity.
- Difficulty breathing due to acute bronchoconstriction in severe cases.

Medical treatment

- Corticosteroid inhalers, applied with a specific aerosol chamber for cats, are the treatment of choice.
- Immune therapy by means of a monthly vaccine against the responsible allergens may be successful in a great percentage of cases of asthma.

Recommendations

In order to avoid environmental irritating agents:

- Use clumping litter and discard closed trays with doors.
- Do not smoke or use sprays, incense or aerosol air fresheners.
- Vacuum clean regularly.

CARDIORESPIRATORY SYSTEM

24 Pneumothorax

Accumulation of air in the pleural space, which leads to severe and acute breathing difficulty (dyspnoea).

Types

- **Open:** defect in the thoracic wall, which allows outside air to enter the pleural space.
- **Closed:** air leaks from the lung, bronchi, caudal trachea or oesophagus into the pleural space.
- **Tension:** tear in the pleura, which lets air in at inspiration, but does not let it out at expiration.

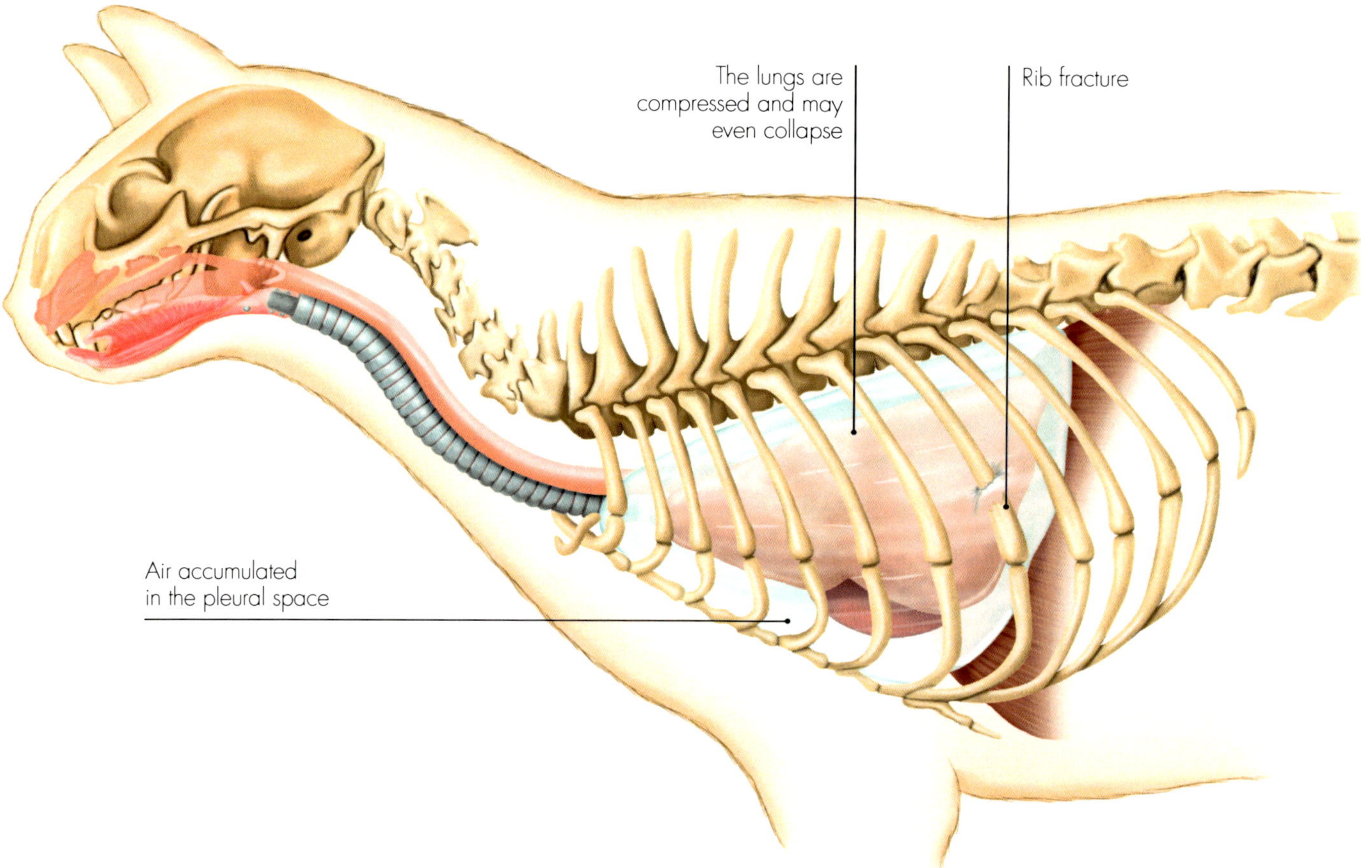

Medical treatment

- Oxygen chamber and analgesic treatment.
- Thoracocentesis and removal of air located in the pleural space.

Surgical treatment

Necessary on very few occasions.

It may be traumatic or spontaneous due to pulmonary disease leading to necrosis of the visceral pleura.

CARDIORESPIRATORY SYSTEM

25 Pleural effusion

It is the presence of fluid in the pleural space, which leads to progressive breathing difficulty.

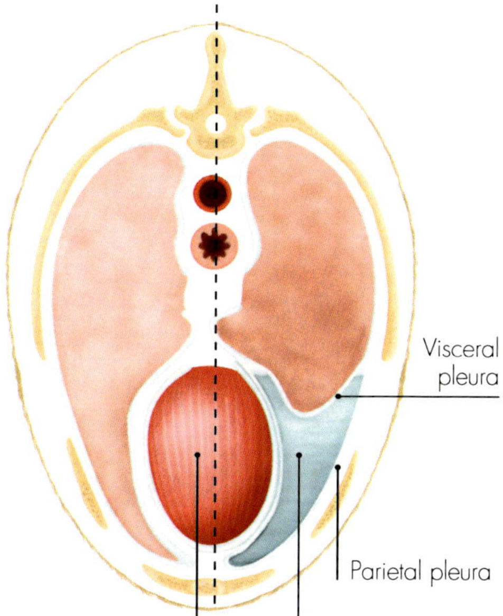

Types of fluid and causes

- **Blood:** trauma, coagulopathies, neoplasms.
- **Chyle:** chylothorax, cardiomyopathy.
- **Non-septic exudate:** FIP, neoplasm, diaphragmatic hernia.
- **Septic exudate:** pyothorax.
- **Transudate:** cardiomyopathy, hypoalbuminaemia, diaphragmatic hernia.

Clinical signs

- Progressive and severe breathing difficulty.

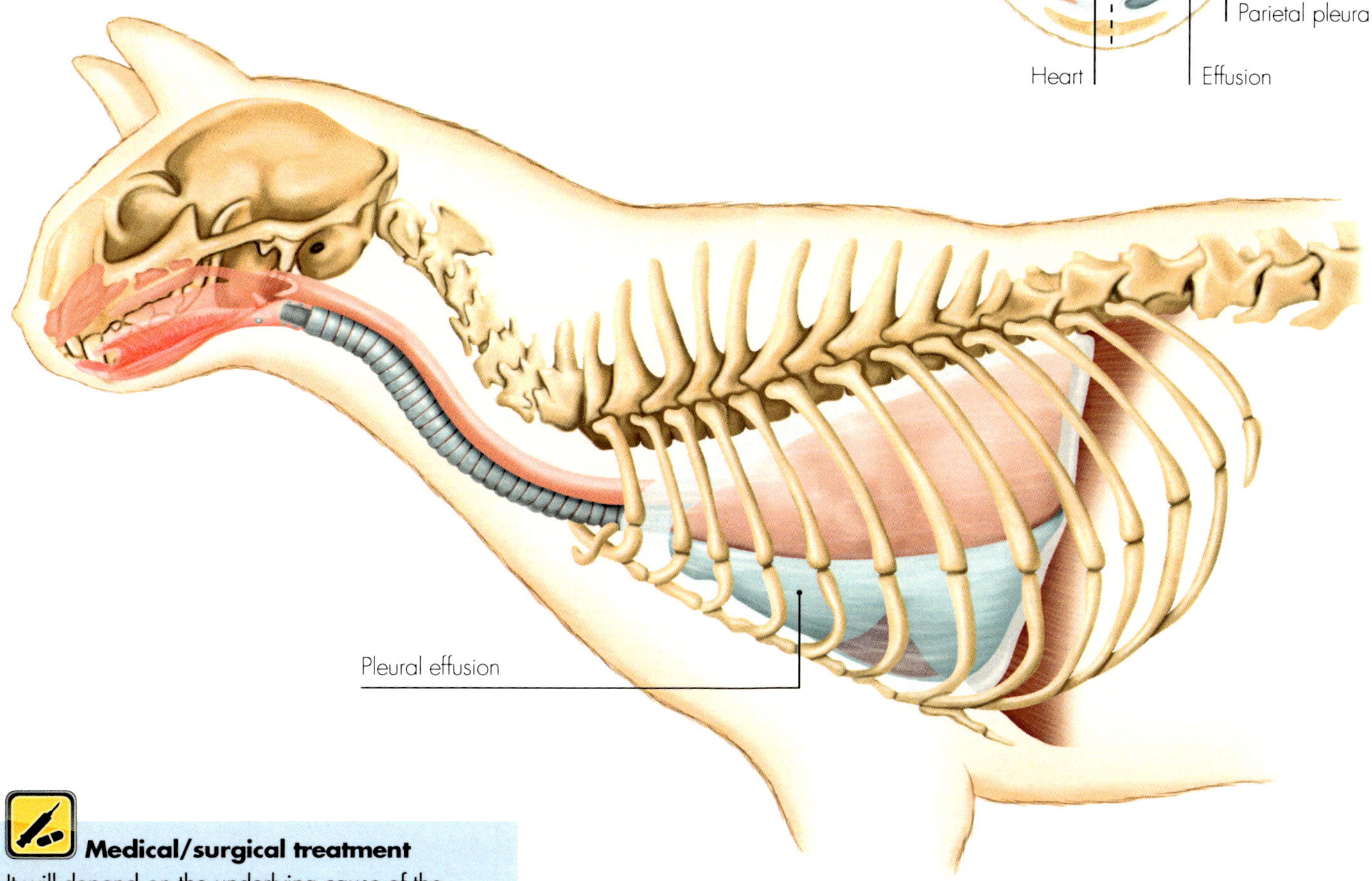

Medical/surgical treatment

It will depend on the underlying cause of the effusion.

The removal of the fluid allows the diagnosis of the cause of the pleural effusion (analysis) and the cat to breathe easily again.

CARDIORESPIRATORY SYSTEM

26 Diaphragmatic hernia

traumatic and peritoneopericardial

Traumatic

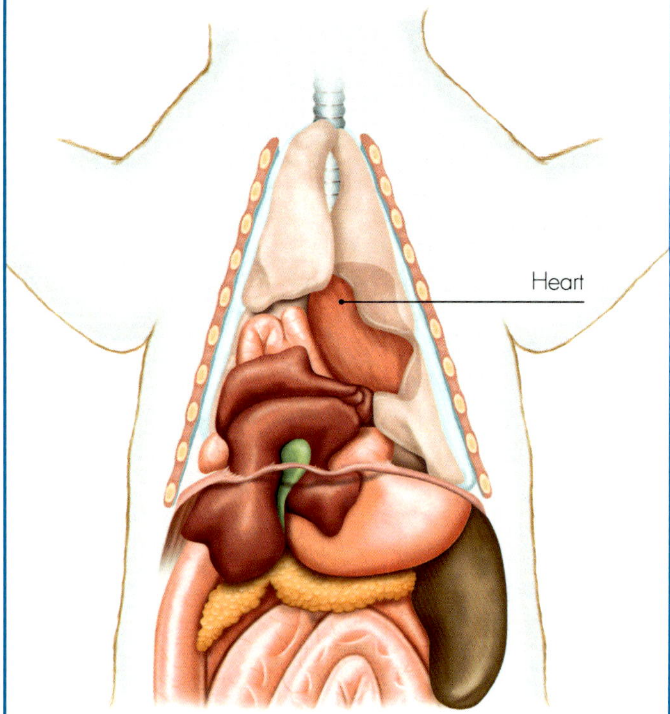

The traumatic rupture of the diaphragm allows the passage of one or various abdominal organs into the thoracic cavity.

- **Causes**: road traffic accidents or high-rise falls.
- **Clinical signs**:
  - Acute form: breathing difficulty and rib cage pain.
  - Chronic form (when it is has not been diagnosed or treated), depending on the herniated abdominal organs:
    - ▷Difficulty breathing with exercise.
    - ▷Depression, anorexia.
    - ▷Digestive signs.

Peritoneopericardial

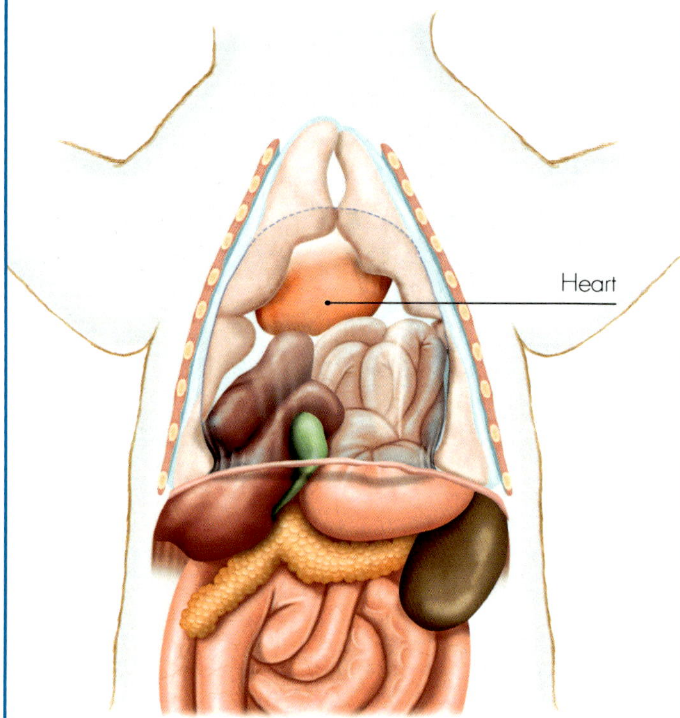

- **Causes**: congenital problem causing the pericardium and peritoneal cavity to be communicated, with the heart permanently surrounded by abdominal structures.
- **Predisposition**: long-haired cats and Himalayans.
- **Clinical signs**:
  - They depend on the herniated organ and on whether it receives appropriate blood supply. It generally affects the liver, small intestine, spleen and stomach.
  - It may be asymptomatic.
  - Gastrointestinal signs and anorexia if it affects the intestine.

Surgical treatment

- To repair the diaphragm.
- In a peritoneopericardial hernia, when it causes clinical symptoms (gastrointestinal obstruction) or when the blood flow to abdominal organs is altered.
- If a hepatic lobe or part of the abdominal fat is herniated, and there are no clinical signs, surgery may be required.

ENDOCRINE SYSTEM

27 Hyperthyroidism

Uncontrolled production of thyroid hormones, thyroxine (T_4) and triiodothyronine (T_3), by the thyroid gland, either due to nodular hyperplasia or to a benign adenoma, although 1 % of the affected animals will develop thyroid carcinoma.

Risk factors

- Cats > 6 years old.
- Goitrogenic substances present in easy-open tins and in additives contained in fish-based or liver-based wet food.
- Diets with very variable iodine concentrations (from deficient to excessive).

Clinical signs

- Unilateral or bilateral nodule in the cervical region (80-90 % of cases).
- Progressive loss of weight, polyphagia, hyperactivity.
- Digestive: chronic vomiting, diarrhoea.
- Cardiac: hypertension, hypertrophic cardiomyopathy.
- Hepatic: increased hepatic enzyme levels.

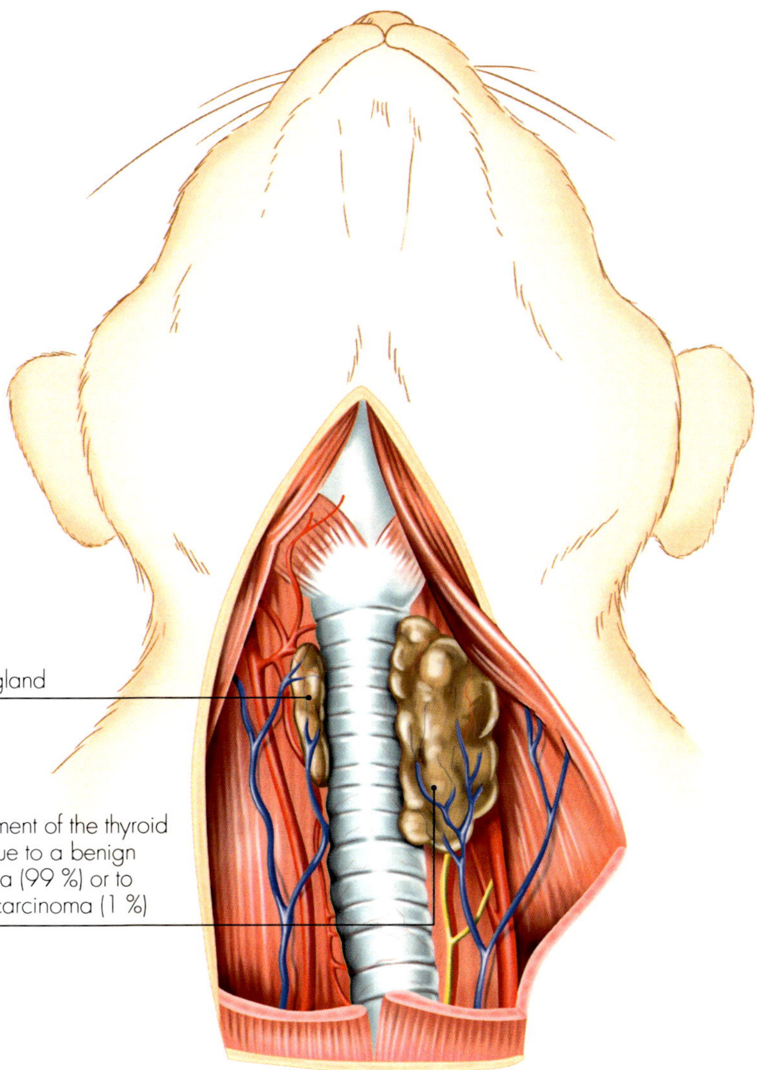

It is the most frequent endocrine disease in cats.

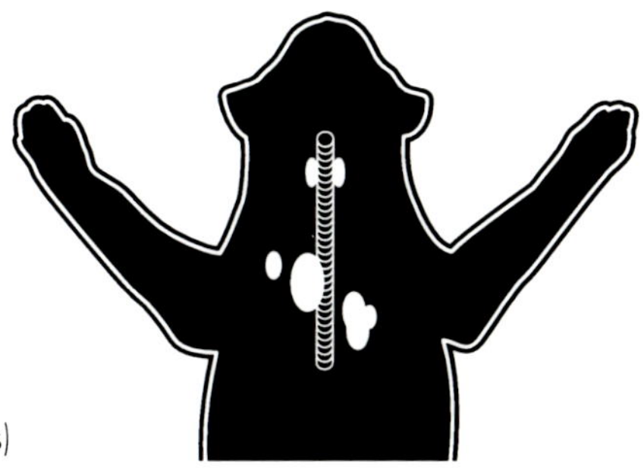

Ectopic thyroid tissue (20% of hyperthyroid cats)

Medical treatment

- Antithyroid drugs.
- Radioactive therapy (iodine 131).

Surgical treatment

Surgical removal (thyroidectomy) in cats with no occult renal disease.

Dietary treatment

Specific diet for the treatment of hyperthyroidism.

ENDOCRINE SYSTEM

28 Feline diabetes

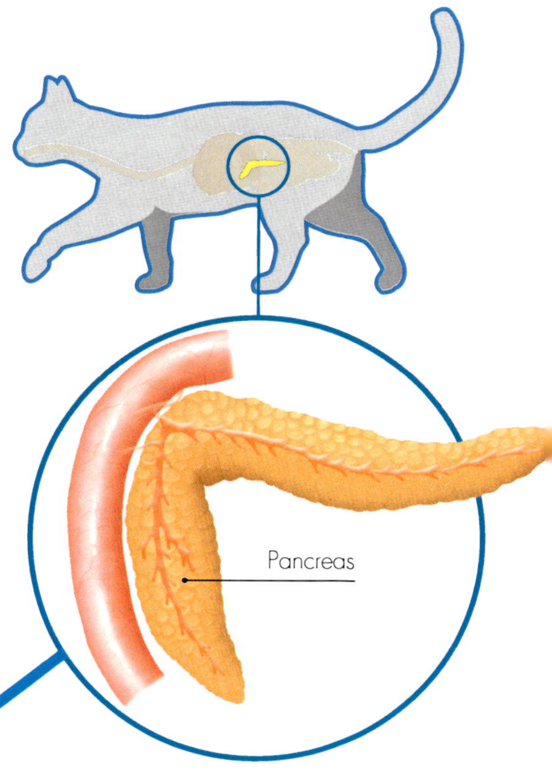

Risk factors

- Age: most diagnosed cats are > 6 years old (greater incidence: 10-13 years of age).
- Breed: Burmese cats have a greater predisposition.
- Inactivity: very frequent in indoor cats.
- Obesity: it is the most important factor, especially in males.
- Infections and inflammations: periodontal disease, infections of the urinary tract, pyoderma, pancreatitis, etc.
- Treatment with corticosteroids or progestogens.

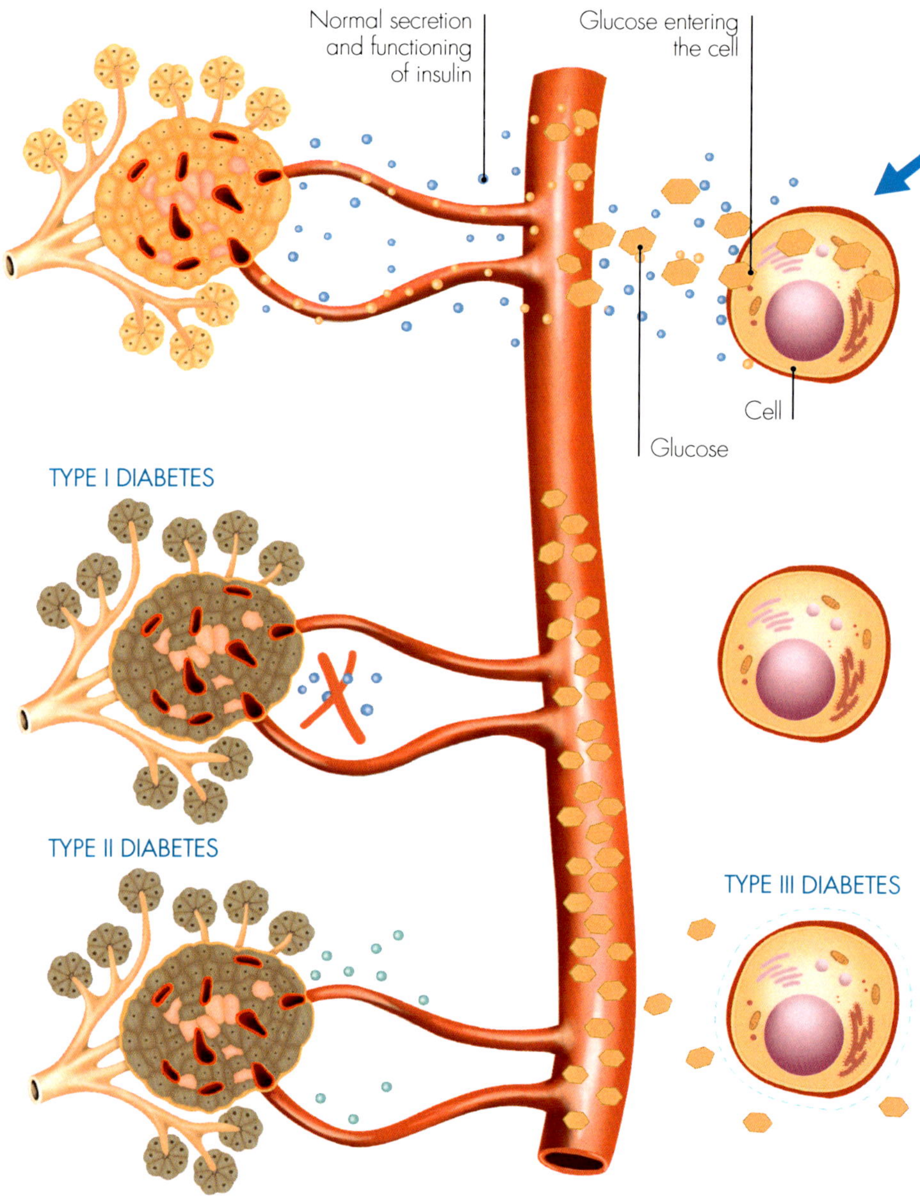

Recovery occurs in up to 67 % of the cats treated with insulin and a specific diet for diabetic cats rapidly after the diagnosis.

Clinical signs

- Polyuria/polydipsia.
- Polyphagia (they eat more).
- Loss of weight.
- Diabetic neuropathy: hind limb weakness and in acute cases, of the forelimbs too.

TYPE I DIABETES: destruction of the pancreatic cells by the immune system.

TYPE II DIABETES: combination of an inappropriate secretion of insulin and resistance to its action in tissues (due to obesity, infection, etc.).

TYPE III DIABETES: due to diseases that lead to high resistance to the action of insulin: hyperadrenocorticism, acromegaly, pancreatitis, pancreatic adenocarcinoma, administration of glycocorticoids, etc.

ENDOCRINE SYSTEM

29 Obesity

Obesity is a serious disease that must be treated with diet and lifestyle changes.

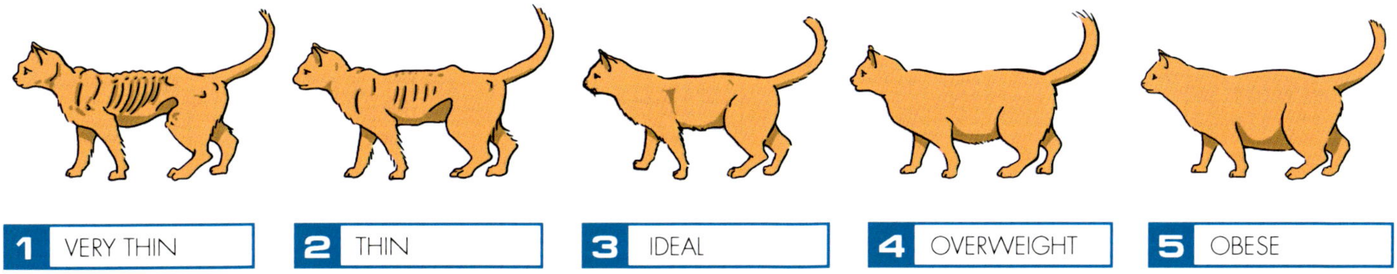

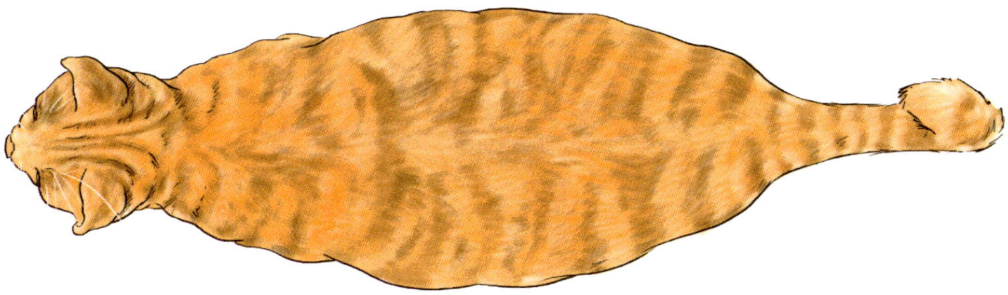

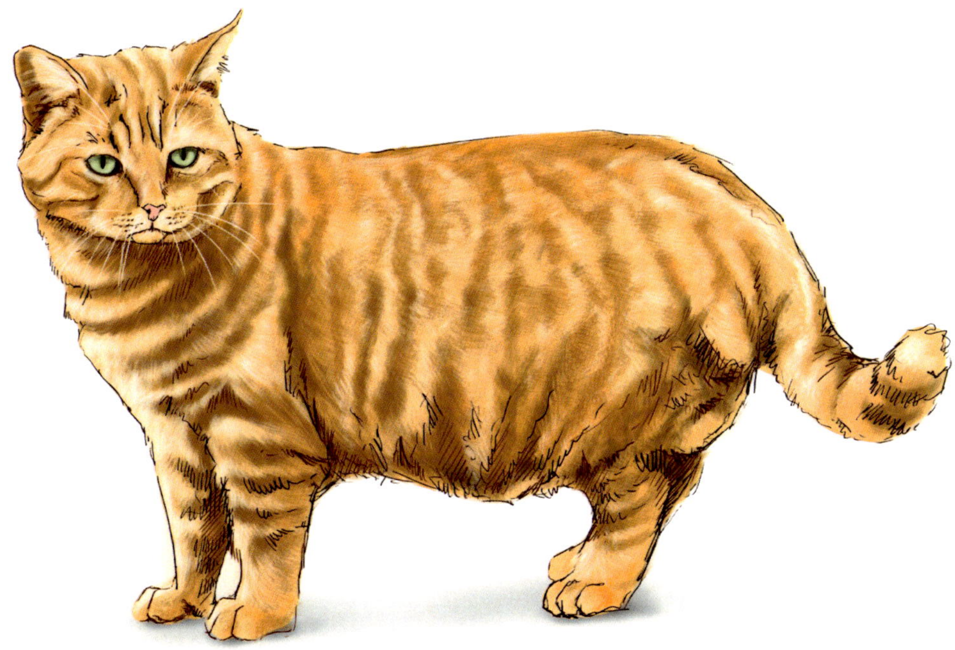

Risk factors

- Neutering: it reduces the energy needs of cats by 20 %.
- Inactivity: frequent in indoor cats.
- Age: cats between 2 and 10 years old are the most prone to it.
- Feeding: food with a high calorie content and great palatability.

Obesity increases the risk of suffering from certain diseases.

Associated complications

- Diabetes mellitus.
- Osteoarthritis.
- Hepatic lipidosis.
- Skin alterations.
- Respiratory problems.
- Dystocia.
- Intolerance to exercise.
- Lower immune functions.
- Greater anaesthetic risk.
- Shorter life expectancy.

Dietary treatment

Calorie-restricted diets.

Recommendations

Increased daily activity by means of interactive food dispensers and increased daily play (*Nepeta cataria* plant –catnip–, laser pointers, etc.)

SKIN AND ANEXA

30 Structures of the skin in cats

Skin layers

1. Epidermis.
2. Dermis.
3. Subcutaneous tissue or hypodermis.

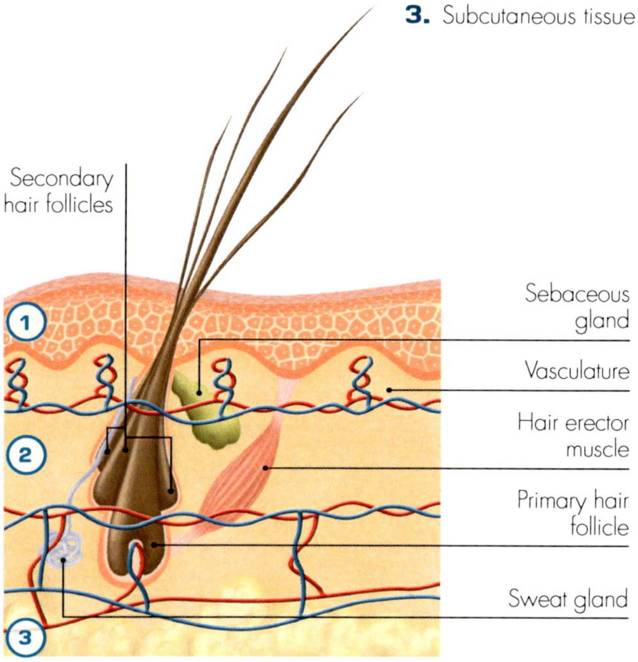

NORMAL HAIR

Hair grows to a certain length, which varies depending on the body region and is genetically predetermined.

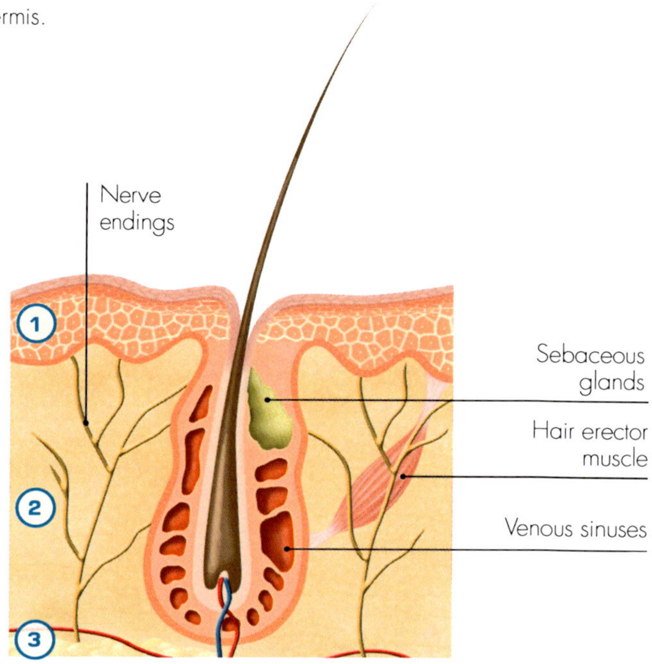

TACTILE HAIR OR VIBRISSA

- They are located on each side of their nose, above their eyes, below their ears (angle of the mandible) and at the back of their carpus.
- They are very sensitive to pressure or to air currents.

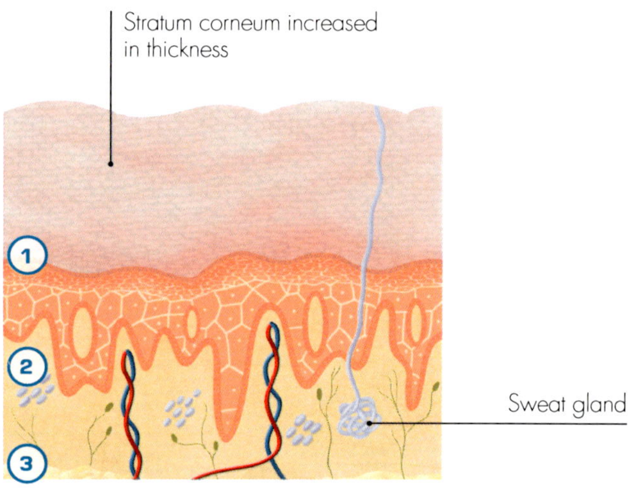

PAW PAD

- Protective tissue of the paws that also provides cushioning.
- They secrete pheromones through sweat.

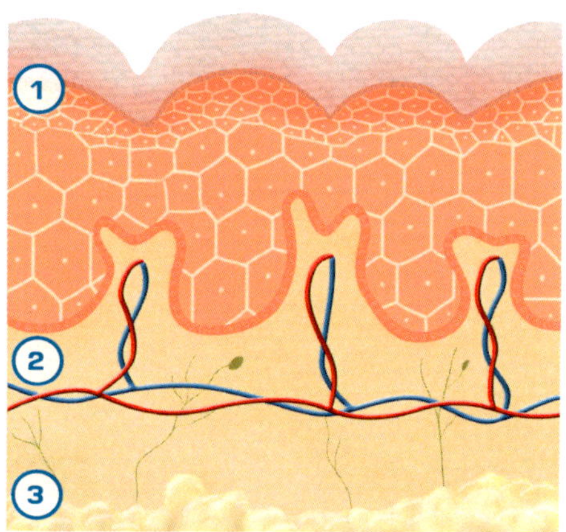

NASAL EPITHELIUM

- It may have different colours depending on the cat's breed and coat.
- Its temperature and degree of humidity are not always an indication of the cat's state of health.

SKIN AND ANEXA

31 Characteristics of claws

Disorders of claws

- Macronychia: abnormally long claws.
- Onychalgia: pain in the claws.
- Onychoclasis: breaking of claws.
- Onychocryptosis (onyxis): ingrown claws.
- Onychodystrophy: abnormal claw formation.
- Onychogryphosis: hypertrophy and abnormal curvature of claws.
- Onychomadesis: sloughing of claws.
- Onychomalacia: softening of claws.
- Onychorrhexis: longitudinal striations and breaking of claws.
- Onychoschizia: splitting or lamination of claws.
- Onychia (onychitis): inflammation of part of the claw.
- Paronychia: inflammation/infection of the folds of tissue surrounding the claw.

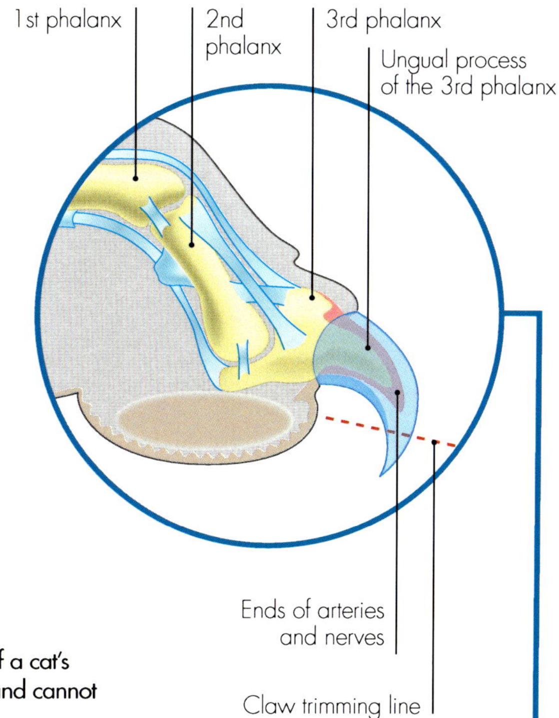

Scratching is part of a cat's natural behaviour and cannot be eliminated.

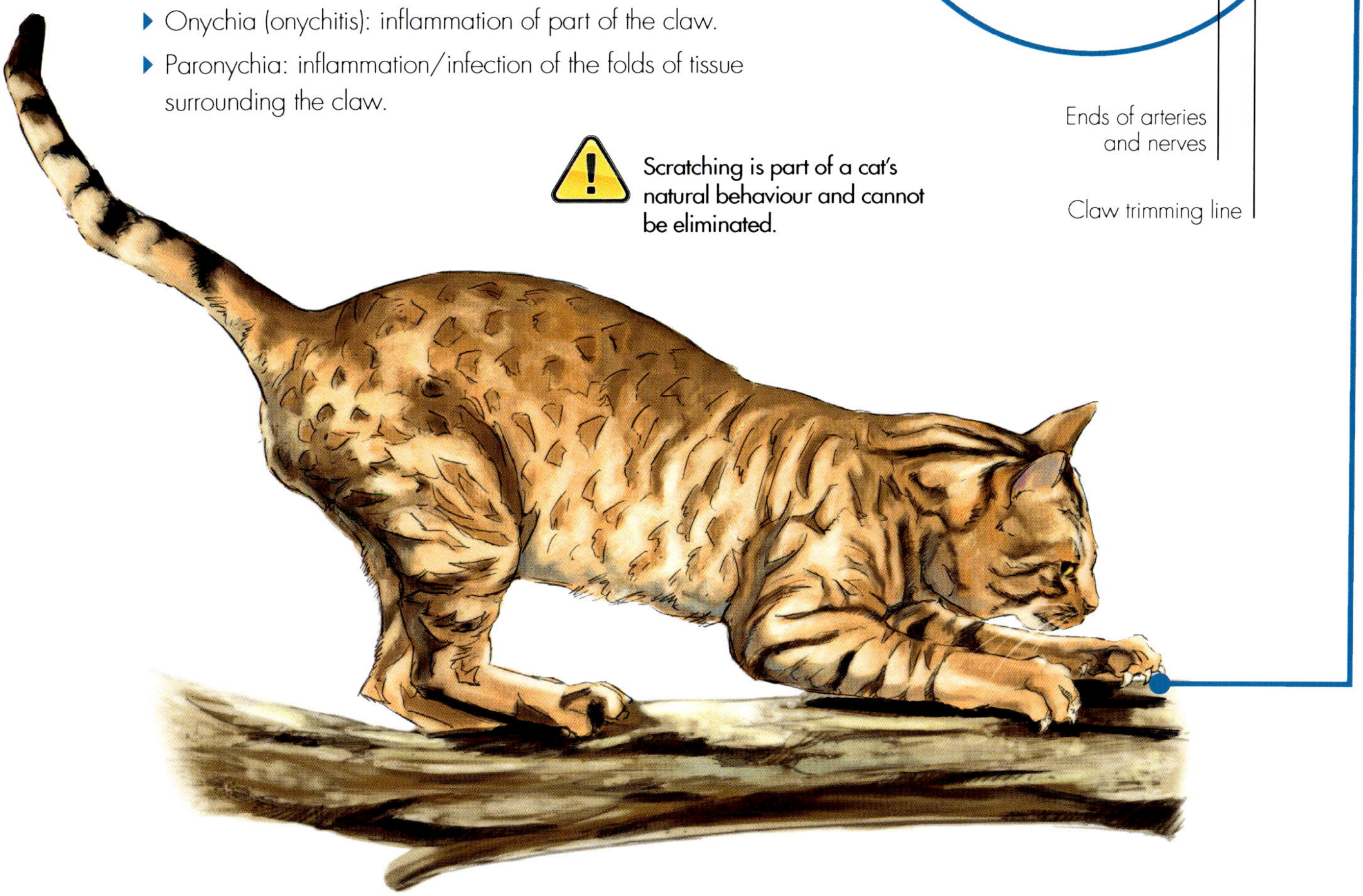

Recommendations

To prevent a cat form scratching sofas or other furniture, the following should be done:

- Place a scratcher in the area where the cat usually rests.
- Scratchers should be sturdy and not wobble when scratched. Scratching posts are ideal.
- If the cat already scratches a sofa or other surface, this latter should be cleaned and an adequate scratching post should be placed next to it.
- A cat should not be forced to use a scratcher. Instead, play should be used to encourage the cat to scratch it.

SKIN AND ANEXA

32 Feline acne

An increase in the activity of the sebaceous glands in the chin leads to the formation of blackheads, which are particularly noticeable in pale-coloured cats.

The diagnostic tests are: cutaneous cytology, skin scraping, biopsy and bacterial and fungal cultures.

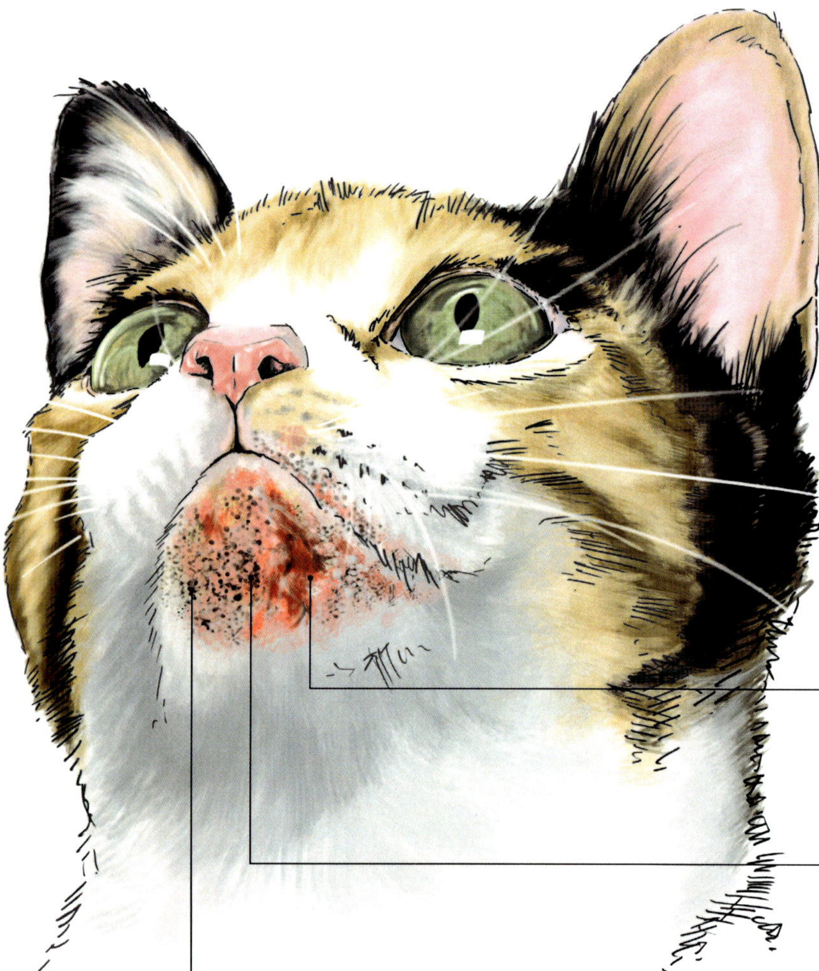

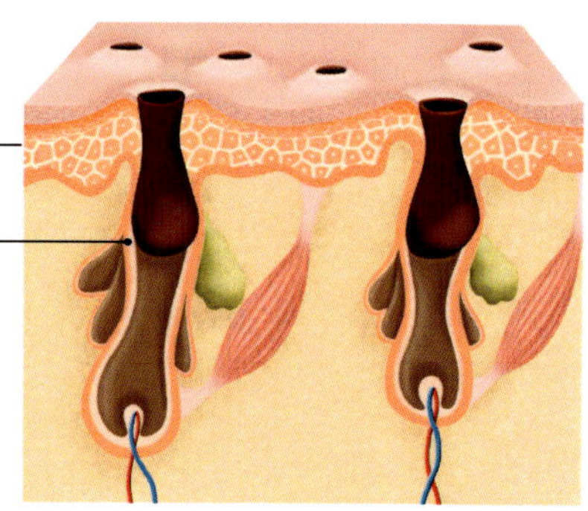

Triggering factors

Multifactorial process:

- Greater production of fat.
- Immunosuppression and stress.
- Respiratory viruses (whether they are direct causative agents or responsible for immunosuppresion and stress is under research).
- Bacterial overgrowth.

Medical treatment

Depending on the severity, the administration of a combination of drugs (antibiotics, antifungal medication, corticosteroids, essential fatty acids, etc.) by oral and topical routes will be required.

Clinical signs

- Blackheads on the chin, upper lip and labial commissure.
- If it worsens, erythema, pustules and even firm and inflamed nodules (furunculosis) will appear. Abscesses in very severe cases.
- Itching in case of bacterial infection.

SKIN AND ANEXA

33 Feline hypersensitivity

Allergies

Hypersensitivity is an excessive and inappropriate immune response to usually harmless allergens. It leads to skin and sometimes digestive disorders.

Clinical signs

Itching associated with one or various patterns of reaction:

- Symmetrical alopecia.
- Miliary dermatitis.
- Eosinophilic granuloma complex.
- Pruritus on the face and neck.

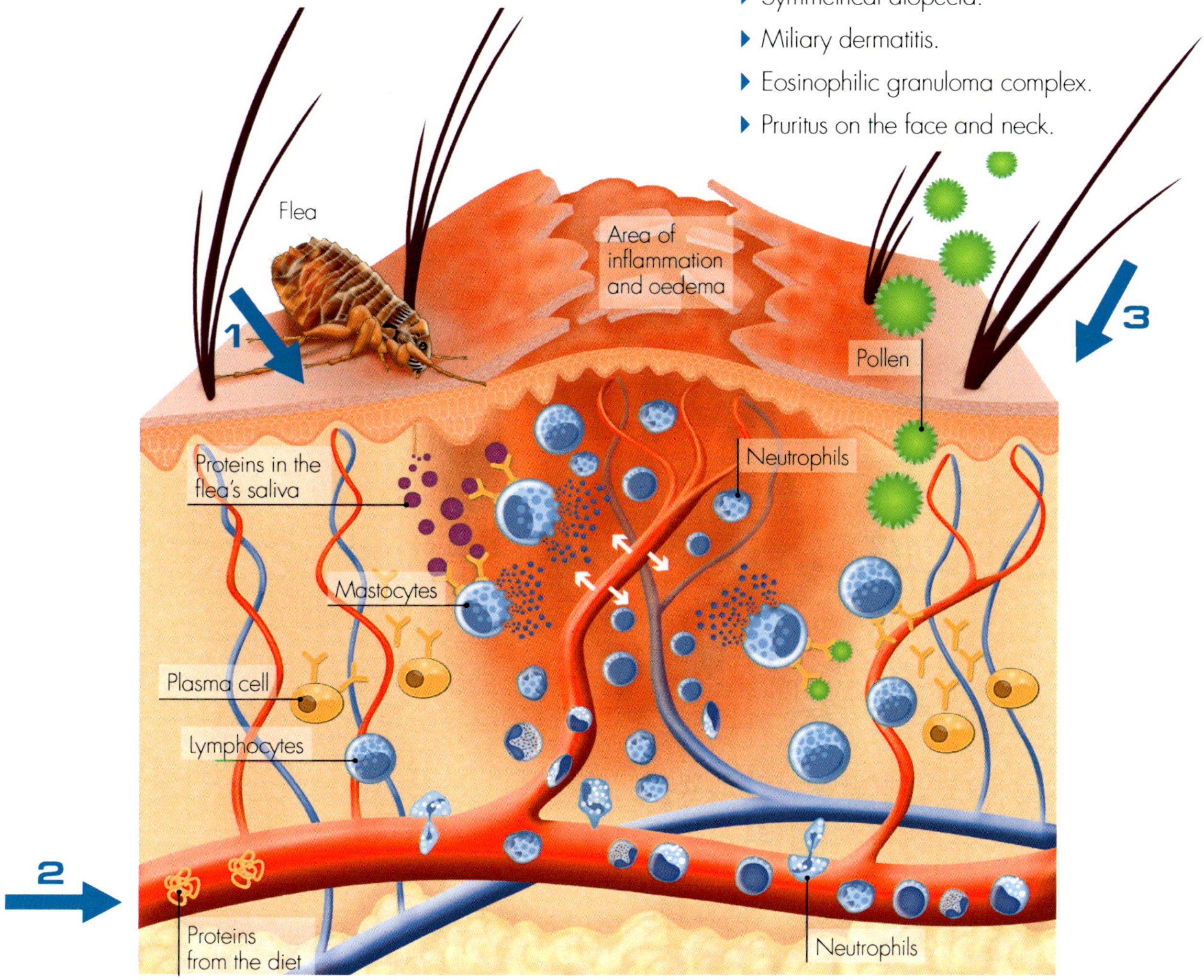

1 Hypersensitivity to flea bites

- Fleas release substances that cause inflammatory reactions at the bite site.
- It is the first cause of hypersensitivity to rule out.
- Treatment: adulticides together with products to control larvae and eggs in the environment.

2 Adverse reaction to food

- Cats between 3 months and 12 years of age.
- Cutaneous and/or digestive clinical signs. Less frequent: interdigital erythema, acne, pododermatitis, conjunctivitis and angioedema.
- Allergens: fish, dairy products, beef, chicken, lamb, gluten, additives, corn and rice.
- Treatment: diet excluding the foods the cat is allergic to.

3 Atopic dermatitis

- Cats between 6 months and 3 years of age.
- Otitis, pododermatitis and seborrheic alterations may be observed together with pruritus and the aforementioned patterns of reaction.
- Allergens: dust mites and pollens.
- Treatment: immunotherapy with hyposensitisation vaccines (70-80 % efficacy).

SKIN AND ANEXA

34 Feline eosinophilic granuloma complex

The eosinophilic granuloma complex is a cutaneous reaction pattern caused by hypersensitivity (atopy, adverse reaction to food, hypersensitivity to flea bites). It has three manifestations: indolent ulcer, eosinophilic granuloma and eosinophilic plaque.

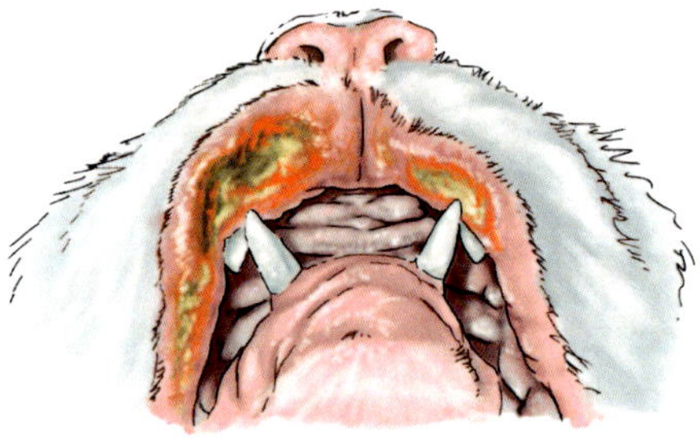

Indolent ulcer

- Ulcerative lesion of the upper lip which can extend to the hard palate.
- It may be uni- or bilateral and, in spite of its appearance, it does not cause pain.

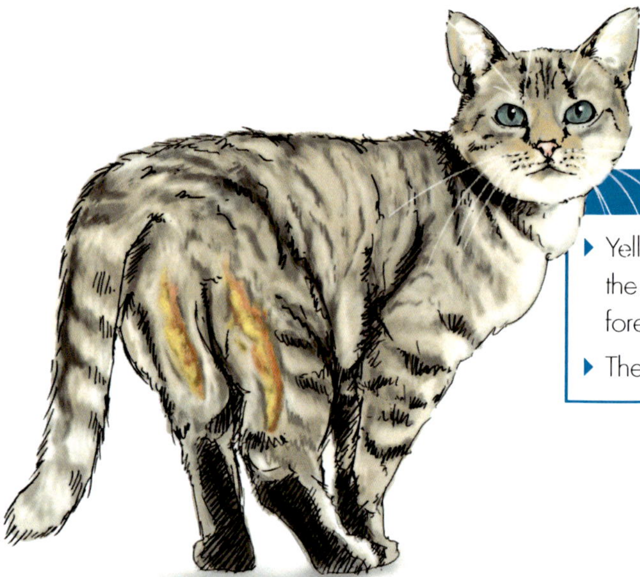

Linear granuloma

- Yellowish to pink linear lesions on the back of one or the two hind legs. It may also appear in the oral cavity, forelimbs and chin (chin oedema).
- There is no associated pruritus or pain.

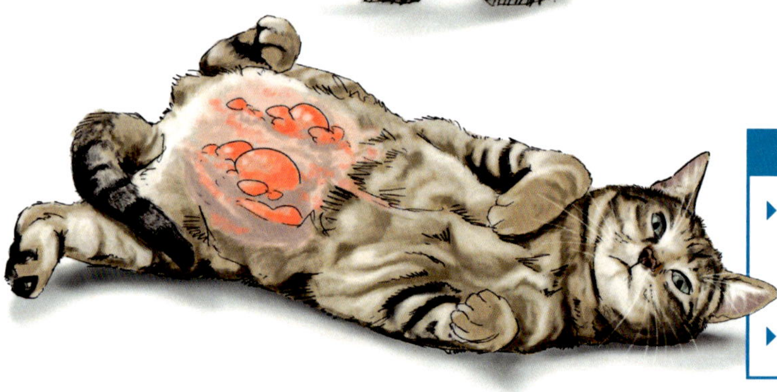

Eosinophilic plaque

- Erythematous (reddish) and ulcerated lesions in the form of a plaque and located on the abdomen, inner thighs, inguinal region, neck and interdigital spaces.
- Pruritus is severe.

Medical treatment

The definitive treatment involves the diagnosis of the cat's hypersensitivity.

SKIN AND ANEXA

35 Alopecia

The new clinical approach to alopecia is to first observe its distribution pattern and then the lesions that accompany the alopecia.

Clinical approach to alopecia according to distribution patterns			
Focal o multifocal	Irregular	Regional	Generalised
• Demodicosis • Superficial pyoderma • Dermatophytosis • Alopecia areata • Cutaneous asthenia • Traction alopecia • Inflammatory reaction at the site of injection • Cicatricial alopecia	• Demodicosis • Cheyletiellosis • Dermatophytosis • Pediculosis • Rash caused by drugs • Lupus erythematosus • Telogen effluvium • Hyperadrenocorticism	• Lupus erythematosus • Endocrine alopecia • Hyperadrenocorticism • Psychogenic alopecia • Post-clipping alopecia • Alopecia of the ears • Acquired symmetrical alopecia • Paraneoplastic alopecia	• Dermatophytosis • Lupus erythematosus • Reaction to drugs • Alopecia areata • Hypotrichosis • Telogen effluvium
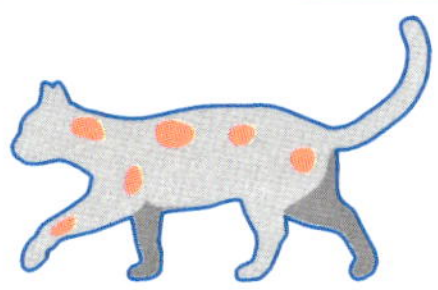	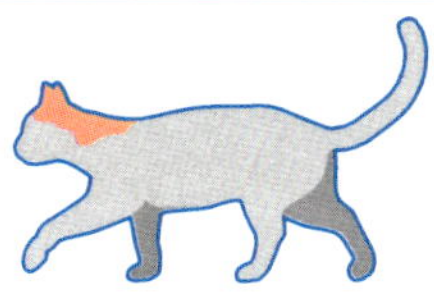	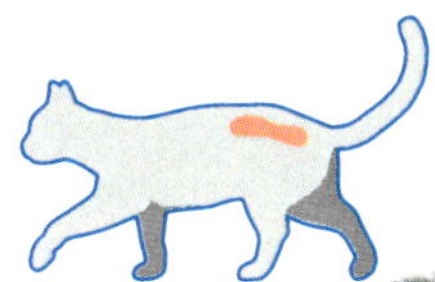	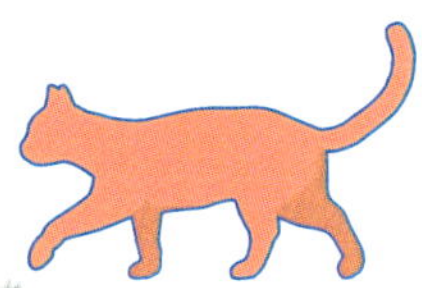

In addition to the focal, multifocal, irregular, regional or generalised absence of hair, alopecia may be accompanied, depending on the cause, by other secondary clinical signs such as pruritus, inflammation, scabs, scaling, pustules, etc.

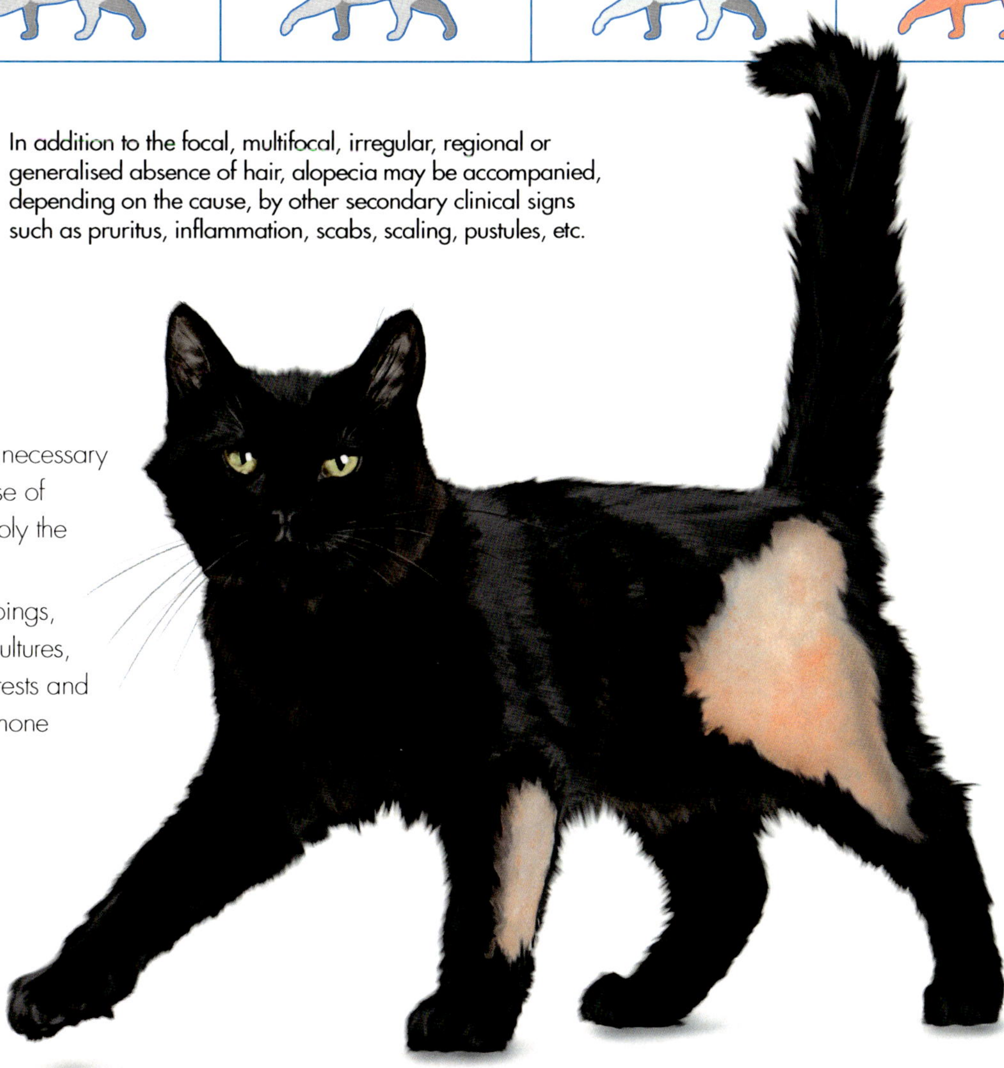

Diagnosis

- Several tests may be necessary to determine the cause of the alopecia and apply the specific treatment.
- Usual tests: skin scrapings, trichograms, fungal cultures, skin biopsies, blood tests and determination of hormone levels.

SKIN AND ANEXA

36 Idiopathic facial dermatitis in Persian cats

Its origin is not well known. It manifests as an abnormally abundant seborrheic discharge, which favours the proliferation of bacteria and yeasts (*Malasezzia*). It usually occurs in cats between 10 months and 6 years of age and must be differentiated from other conditions such as demodicosis, feline acne, dermatophytosis and hypersensitivity.

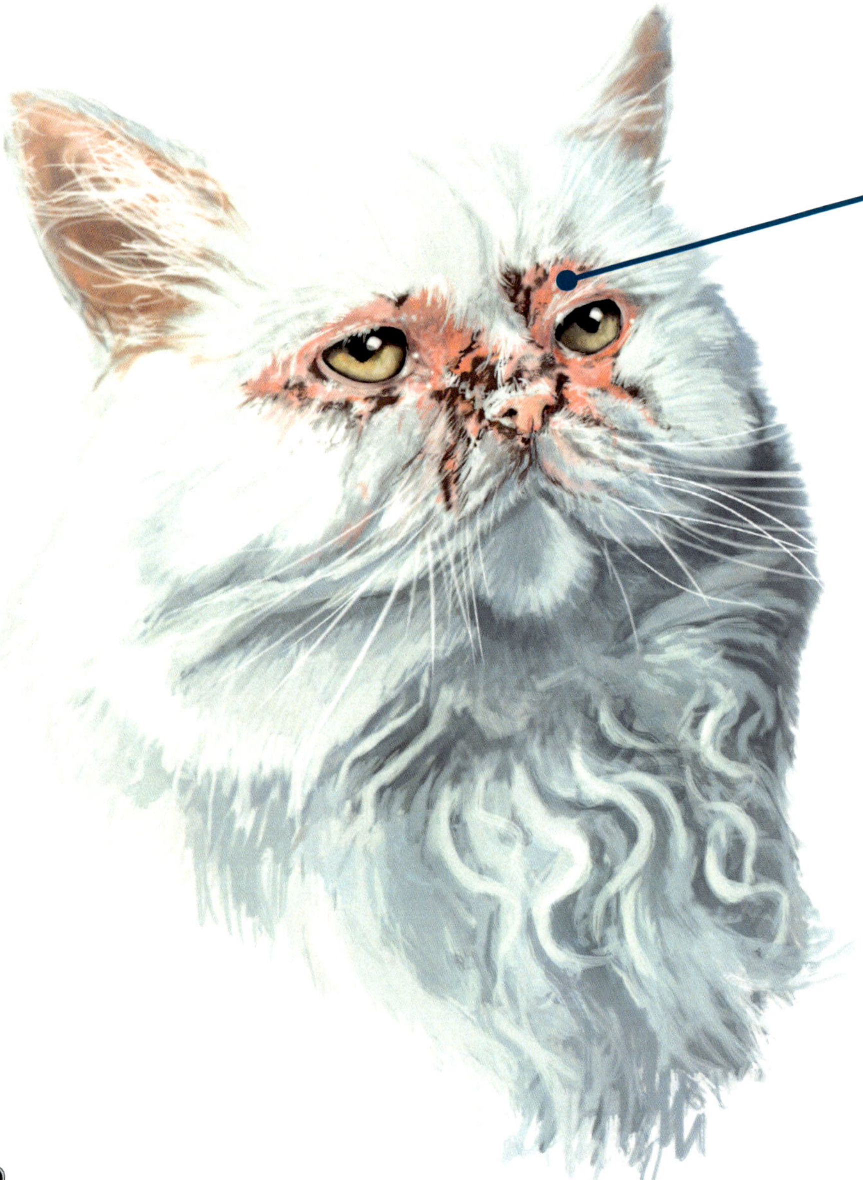

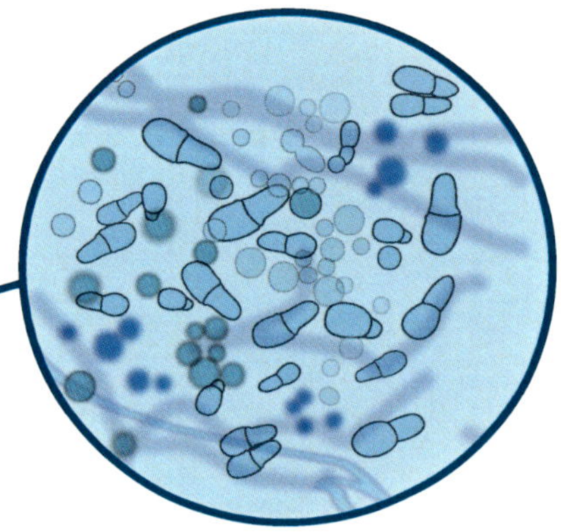

As the cause of this disease is still unknown, there is no completely effective treatment available.

Clinical signs

- Accumulation of black, waxy and very adhering material which causes matting of the hair on the cat's chin and periocular skin folds ("dirty face syndrome").
- Variable erythema (reddening) in the affected regions.
- In many cases, bilateral erythematous dermatitis.
- Complication with the growth of bacteria and *Malassezia*.
- Submandibular lymphadenopathy (occasionally).

Medical treatment

- It focuses on controlling infections caused by bacteria and yeasts with oral products and topical lotions.
- Some cases respond to the use of ciclosporin.

SKIN AND ANEXA

37 Dermatophytosis

It is an infection of the skin, hair and claws caused by the fungi *Microsporum*, *Trochophyton* and *Epidermophyton*.

Disease transmissible to humans (zoonosis).

A cat is not considered cured until at least two negative cultures at a 2-week interval have been obtained. If the results are positive, the medical treatment should be maintained.

Clinical signs

- Focal alopecia, with round lesions on the head, face, and forelimbs.
- Localised lesions that may become generalised.
- Scaling.
- Variable degrees of itching, from non-existent to intense.
- Variable degrees of inflammation.

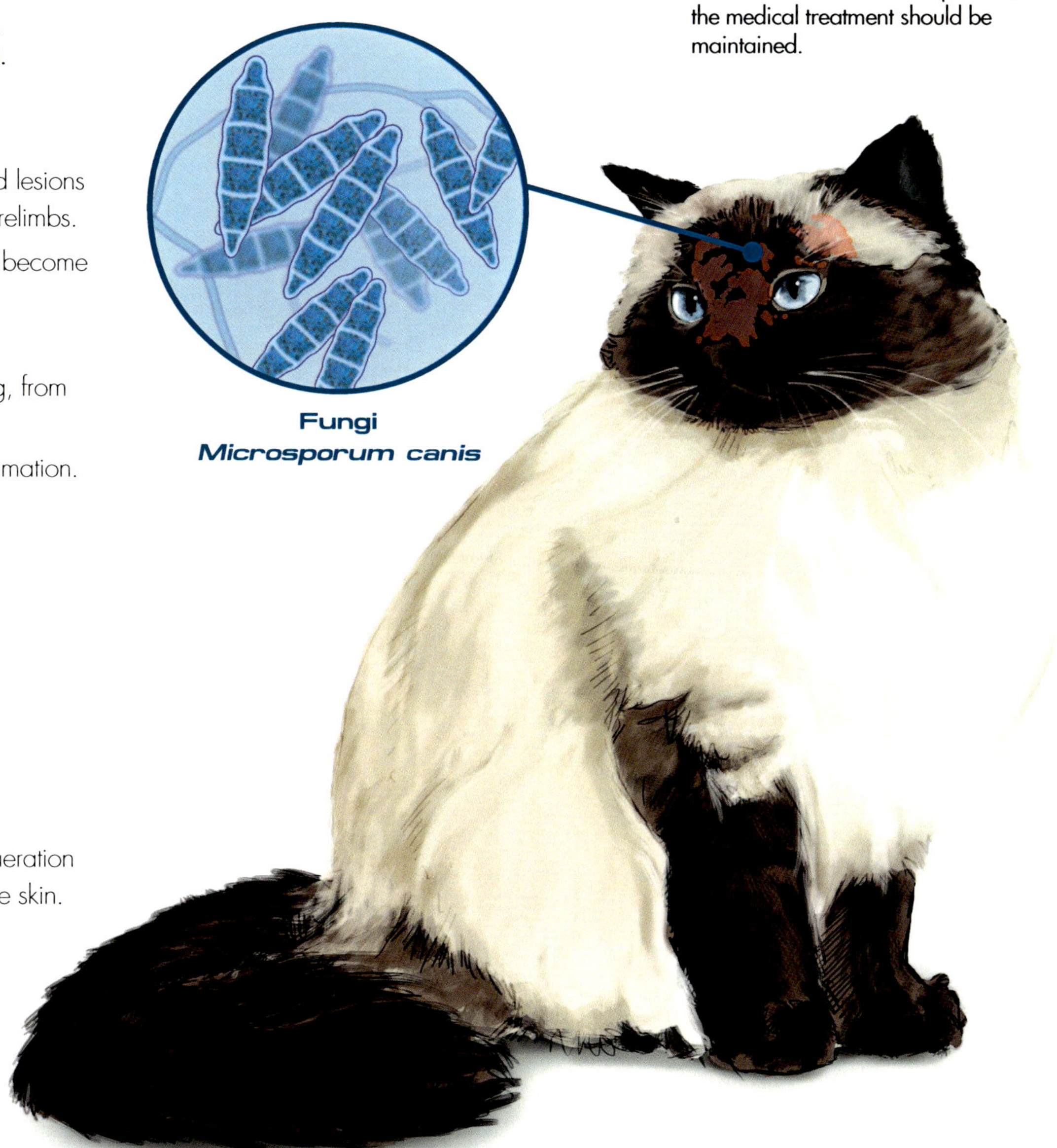

Fungi
Microsporum canis

Predisposing factors

- Cats < 1 year of age.
- Long hair.
- Cats living in groups.
- Immunosuppression.
- Cutaneous trauma, poor aeration or excessive humidity of the skin.

Medical treatment

- Topical: shampoo 2 times/week (reduces environmental contamination).
- Hair clipping 2-3 weeks after starting the oral treatment (reduces environmental contamination and possible reinfections).
- Oral (systemic) treatment with griseofulvin and itraconazole.

Recommendations

- Disinfection of the environment: vacuum clean every day and change the bag frequently.
- Fungicide products are of limited use due to the difficulty in applying them everywhere in the household.

SKIN AND ANEXA

38 Feline notoedric mange

It is caused by the mite *Notoedres cati*. It may affect other animals and people, although it is uncommon.

Notoedres cati burrows into the skin of the cat's face, head and neck to lay its eggs. Mites only survive 48 hours in the environment.

The diagnosis is made by skin scrapings.

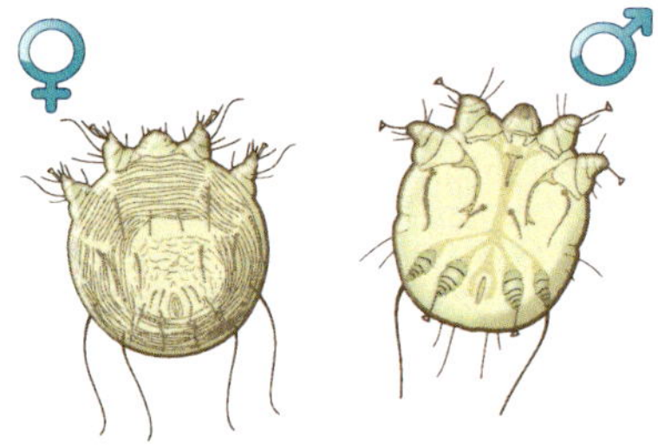

Notoedres cati mites

Young or debilitated cats are the most affected.

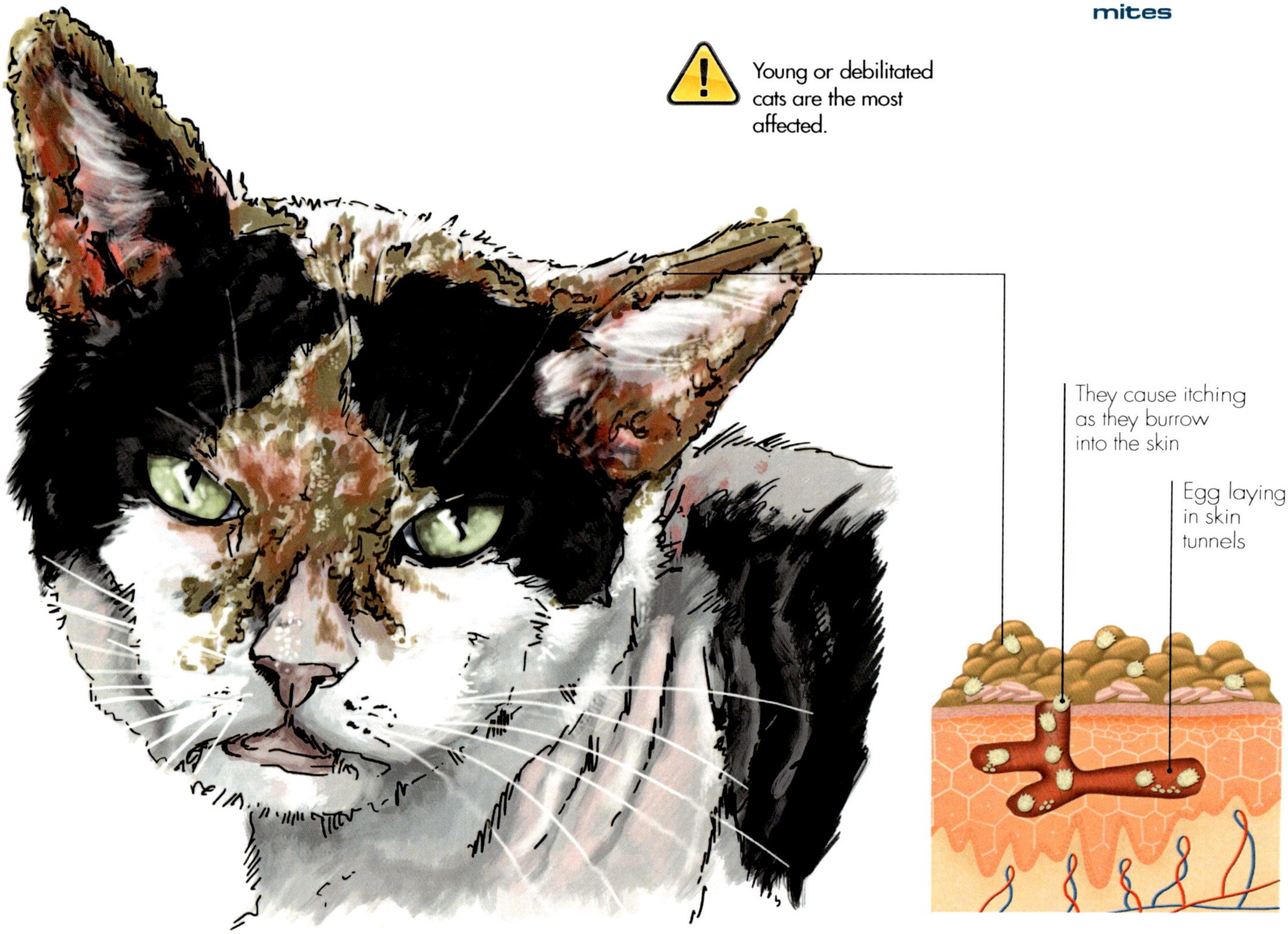

Clinical signs

- Lesions at the tip of the ears, which later extend to the face, head and neck.
- The skin is thickened and covered in scabs.
- Very intense itching; the lesions caused by scratching may become infected.
- Grooming may lead to mites extending to the perineal region and limbs.

Medical treatment

- Requires the use of antiparasitic drugs such as ivermectin and selamectin.
- All the animals in contact with the affected cat must be treated.

SKIN AND ANEXA

39 Otitis caused by *Otodectes cynotis*

The mite *Otodectes cynotis* lives mainly in the ear canal and pinna.

It is highly contagious to other cats through direct contact with infected cats or contaminated environments.

All cats living in same household or shelter, boarding kennel, etc. should be treated at the same time.

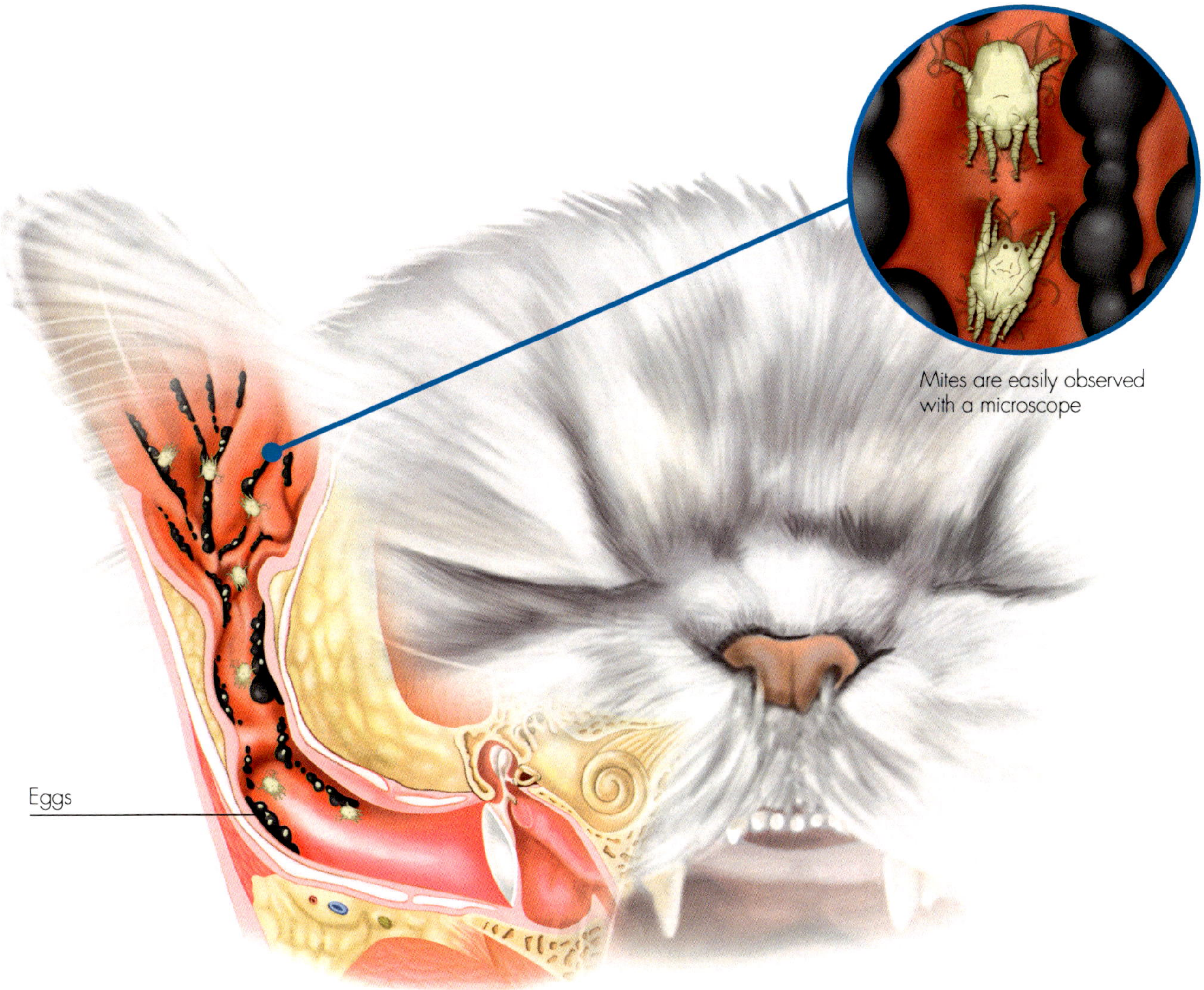

Clinical signs

- Bilateral ceruminous otitis externa.
- Reactions of hypersensitivity with intense itching, lesions caused by scratching and secondary bacterial infections.
- In severe cases, it may cause otitis media.
- Occasionally, lesions on the face and at the tip of the tail.
- Occasional miliary dermatitis.

Medical treatment

- Ear cleaning.
- Topical treatment with ear drops every 12 hours for at least 7 days (their disadvantage is that the rest of the body, where mites may remain, is not treated).
- Administration of a pipette (selamectin, imidacloprid and moxidectin): convenient way of treating the whole cat.

SKIN AND ANEXA

40 Cutaneous tumours

Squamous cell carcinoma and fibrosarcoma

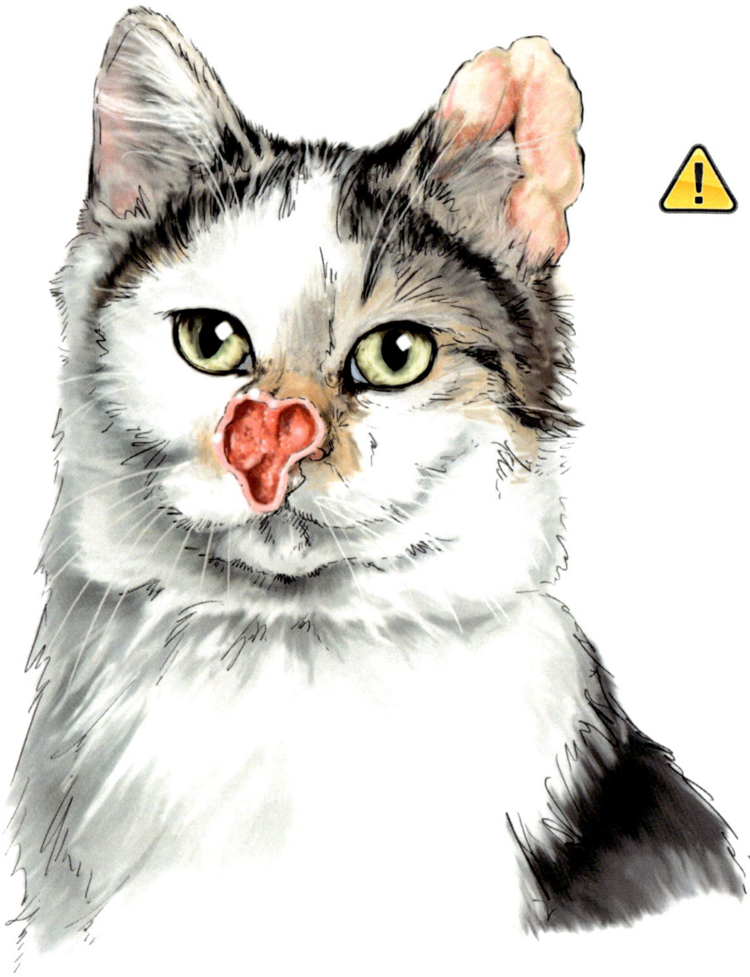

Sun protection is very important in white-haired cats (sun screen, tattooing).

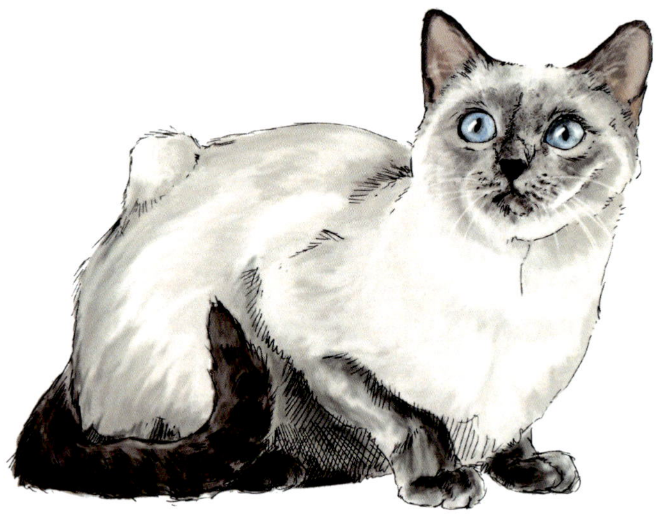

Injection-site fibrosarcoma is caused by an abnormal reaction to chronic inflammation in the tissues of some cats.

Cutaneous squamous cell carcinoma

- It occurs on the nasal plane, eyelids and tip of the ears.
- It is related to prolonged exposure to the sun in pale-coloured cats or in areas with no hair.
- Scabs and ulcerated plaques appear.
- Treatment: surgery, radiotherapy or immunomodulatory therapy depending on the extension and severity.

Fibrosarcoma (injection-site sarcoma)

- It occurs at the site of injection of vaccines, drugs (long-lasting antibiotics, corticosteroids) and other products (non-absorbable sutures, microchip).
- The tumour appears between 1 month and 10 years after the injection.
- It is fast-growing and forms firm and hard nodules.
- Treatment: surgical treatment together with chemotherapy and radiotherapy depending on the extension.

SKIN AND ANEXA

41 Ectoparasites in cats

FLEAS

- Most frequent external parasite in cats.
- They frequently cause allergic dermatitis due to the injection of saliva into their host.
- They can transmit diseases such as feline infectious anaemia.
- They live permanently on the cat.
- A single female can lay up to 50 eggs a day.
- Their eggs fall onto the floor and become larvae, pupae and adult fleas.

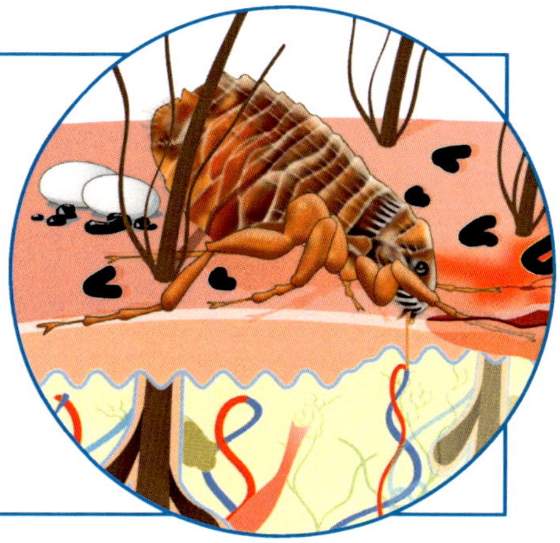

The antiparasitic control of fleas must be carried out both on the cat and on the environment.

TICKS

- They are usually of the genus *Rhipicephalus* (dog tick).
- They may cause local irritation as they inject toxins into their host.
- They transmit diseases (ehrlichiosis, Lyme disease and babesiosis).

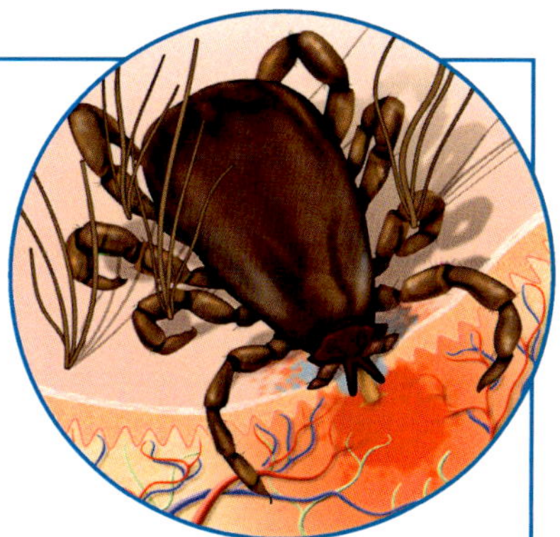

MOSQUITOES

- They bite in areas with less hair: ear margins, on the nose and on the foot pads.
- They frequently cause allergic dermatitis.
- They transmit leishmaniasis and filariasis.

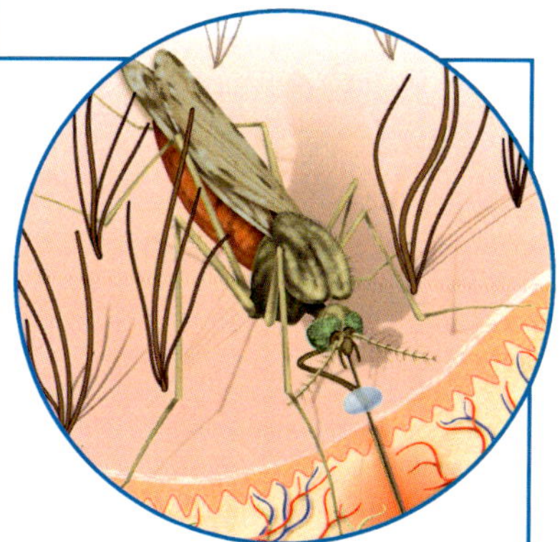

MITES*

- *Demodex cati:* demodectic mange is uncommon in cats. It causes from very mild clinical signs to severe skin disease.
- *Cheyletiella:* is a large and whitish mite, and therefore looks like dandruff.

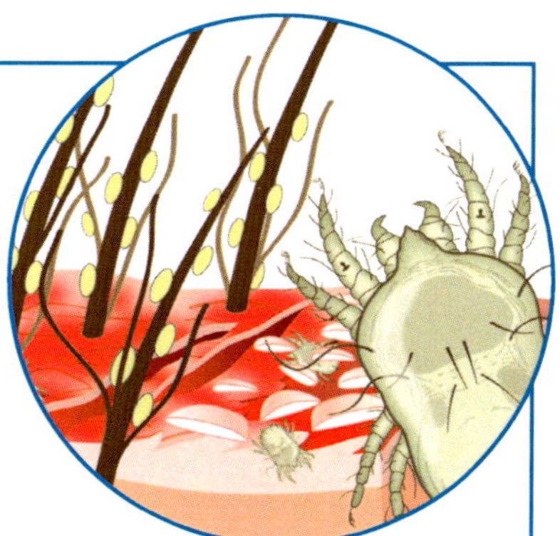

Cheyletiella

LICE

- Cat lice are *Felicola subrostrata* and cannot affect people.
- They are very uncommon.
- They mainly affect kittens living in poor conditions.

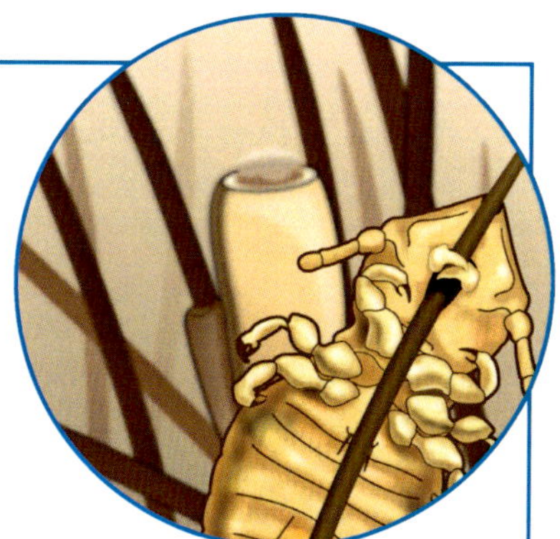

*The mites *Notoedres Cati* and *Otodectes cynotis* are seen in charts 38 and 39 respectively.

DIGESTIVE SYSTEM

42 Teeth in cats

Deciduous and permanent teeth

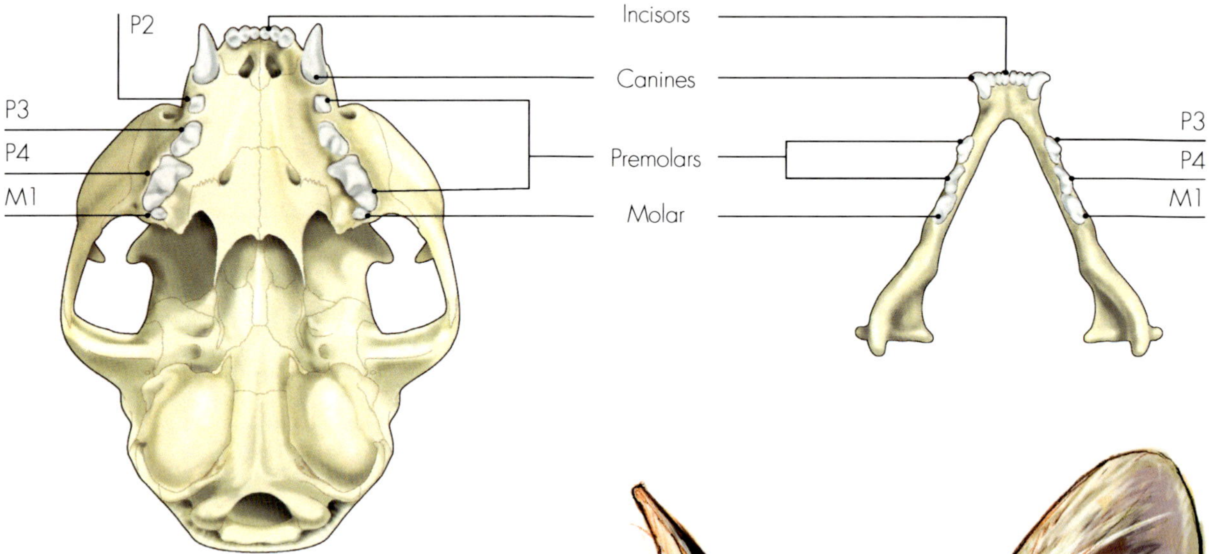

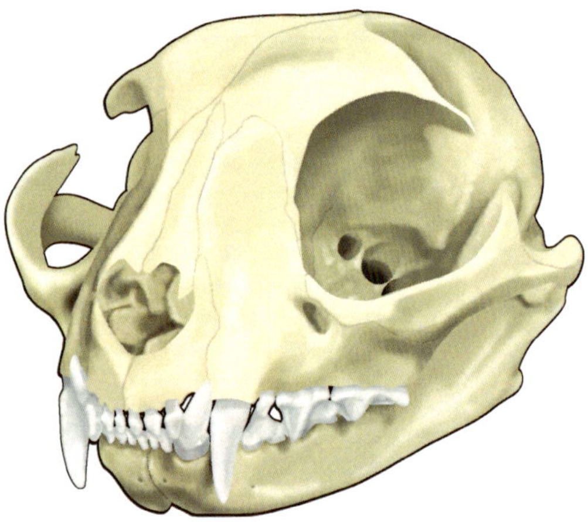

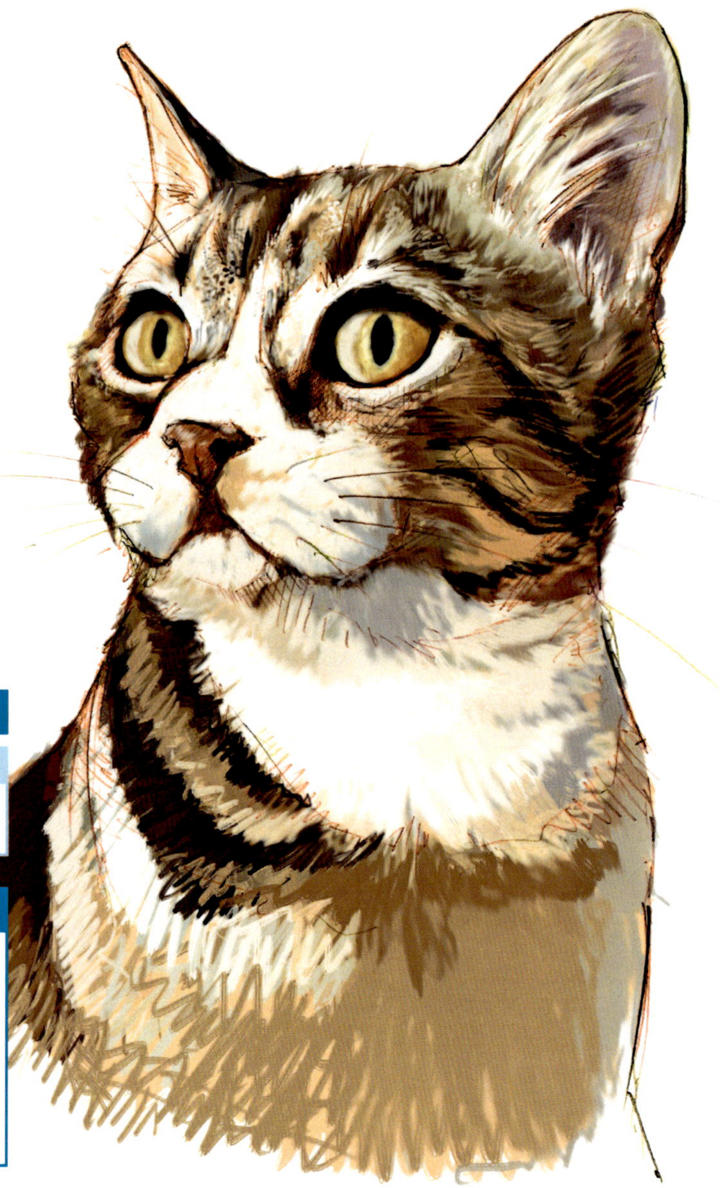

DENTAL FORMULA OF THE CAT	
Deciduous teeth	Permanent teeth
$2 \times \left(I\,\frac{3}{3}\;C\,\frac{1}{1}\;P\,\frac{3}{2} \right) = 26$	$2 \times \left(I\,\frac{3}{3}\;C\,\frac{1}{1}\;P\,\frac{3}{2}\;M\,\frac{1}{1} \right) = 30$

ERUPTION OF PERMANENT TEETH IN THE CAT

- 3.5 - 5.5 months: the milk incisors are replaced by permanent incisors.
- 4 - 5 months: the premolars are replaced.
- 5 - 6 months: eruption of the molars.
- 5.5 - 6.5 months: the canines are replaced.
- 7 months: the permanent dentition is complete.

DIGESTIVE SYSTEM

43 Feline odontoclastic resorptive lesion (FORL)

False caries

It is one of the oral diseases with greater prevalence in cats all around the world. Its cause is still unknown, but it leads to the destruction of the dental tissue in the neck, root and crown of the tooth.

The lesions may be covered by dental plaque or by the inflamed gum, and may therefore go unnoticed. Owners usually do not notice them.

Dental radiographs are essential to determine the exact degree of the lesions.

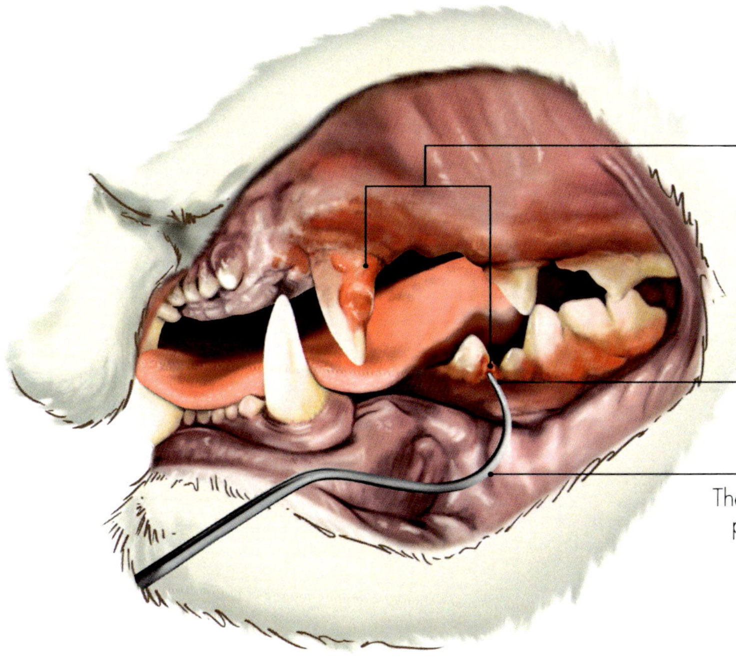

FORL causes pain during mastication. A common reason for the fact that many cats refuse to eat pills is the pain associated with FORL.

Structure of a tooth with FORL

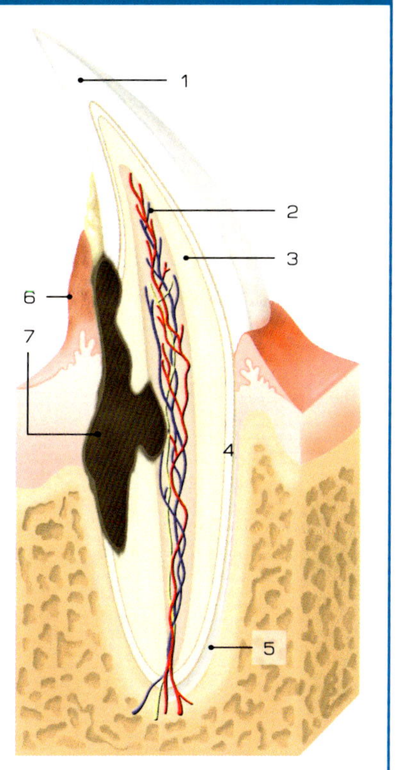

1. Enamel
2. Dental pulp
3. Dentin
4. Cement
5. Periodontal ligament
6. Gingival hyperplasia
7. Dental resorption

Medical treatment

There is no curative or preventive treatment.

Surgical treatment

Extraction is the technique of choice as it eliminates the pain caused by the affected teeth.

Clinical signs

- Changes in the behaviour and in dietary habits (affected cats prefer to eat soft food or stop eating).
- They may drool or show pain (they touch their mouth with their paws).

DIGESTIVE SYSTEM

44 Feline chronic gingivostomatitis

Very painful ulcerative process, which affects all the tissues that are in contact with the saliva and bacterial plaque: gums, mucosae, palatoglossal arch and soft palate.

Diagnosis

- PCR for calicivirus of a sample of oral mucosa.
- Dental radiograph: FORL or periodontal disease.
- Biopsies: only if there is unilateral involvement or proliferation (atypical cases).
- Bacterial culture of the palatoglossal arch in severe cases.

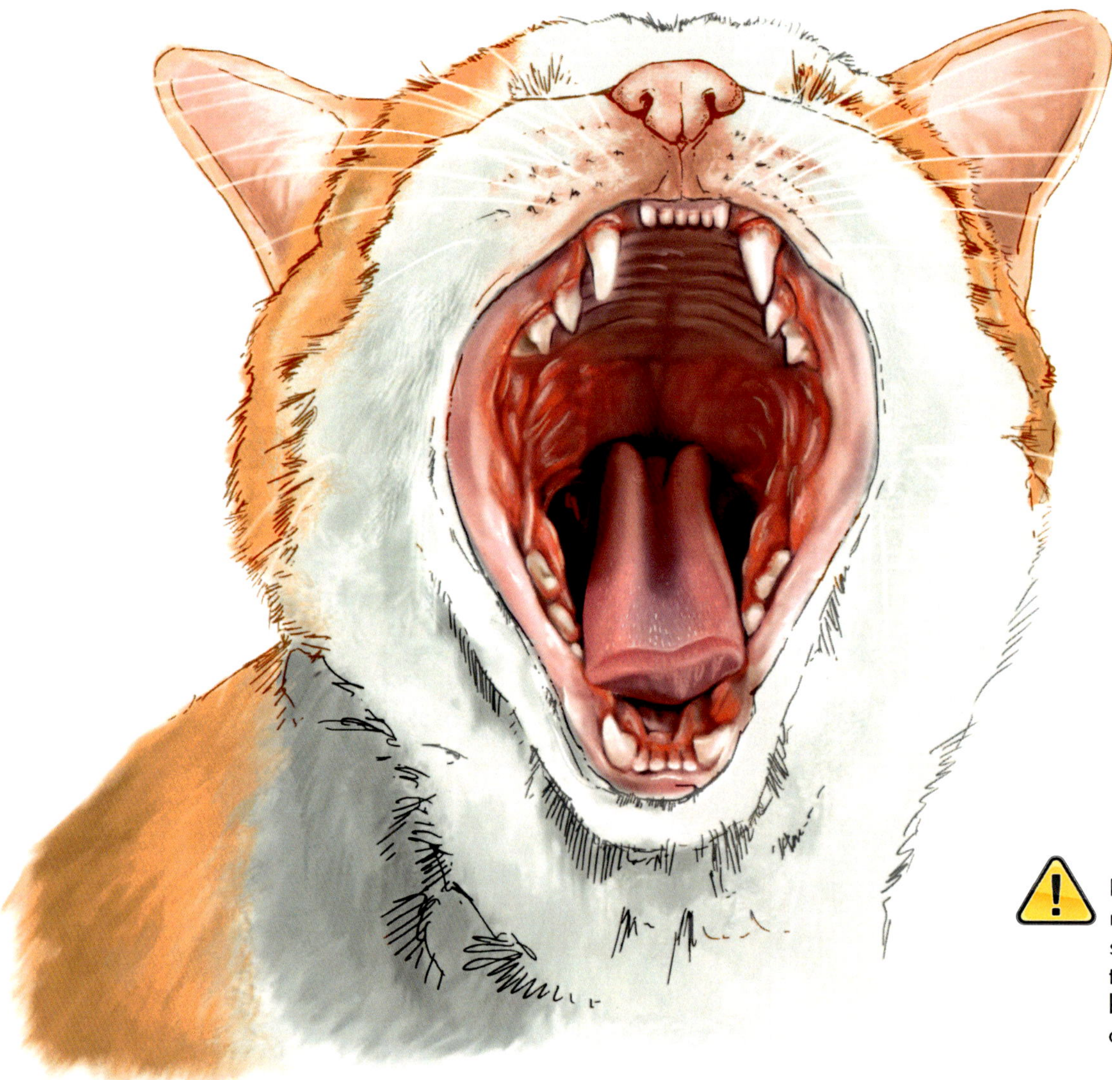

It is due to an exaggerated response of the local immune system to one or several of these conditions: presence of bacterial plaque, periodontal disease, calicivirus, FORL.

Medical/surgical treatment

Varies in function of the cause and severity of the case:

- Pain control: NSAID and opiates.
- Periodontal disease: dental cleaning, extraction of the affected teeth and antibiotic therapy.
- FORL: extraction of the affected teeth.
- Calicivirus: immune modulators.

If there is no response to the treatment, or the clinical picture is initially very severe: extraction of all the teeth (except the canines, if possible), together with analgesics, antimicrobials and immune modulators.

DIGESTIVE SYSTEM

45 Most common feline intestinal parasites

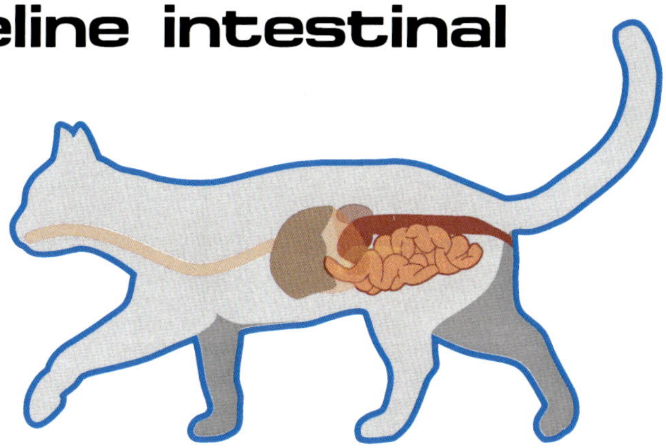

Disease transmissible to humans (zoonosis).

PROTOZOA

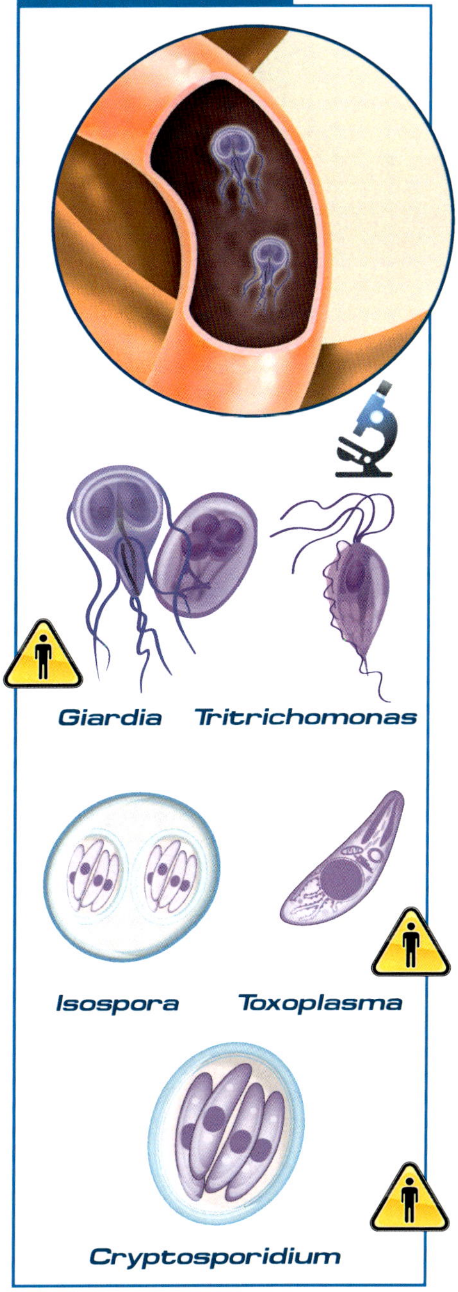

NEMATODES

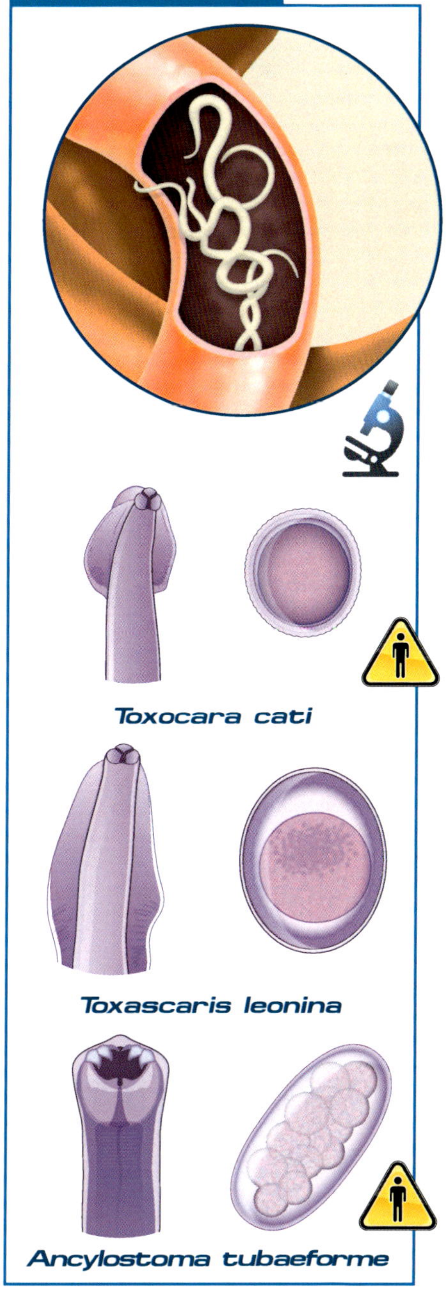

CESTODES

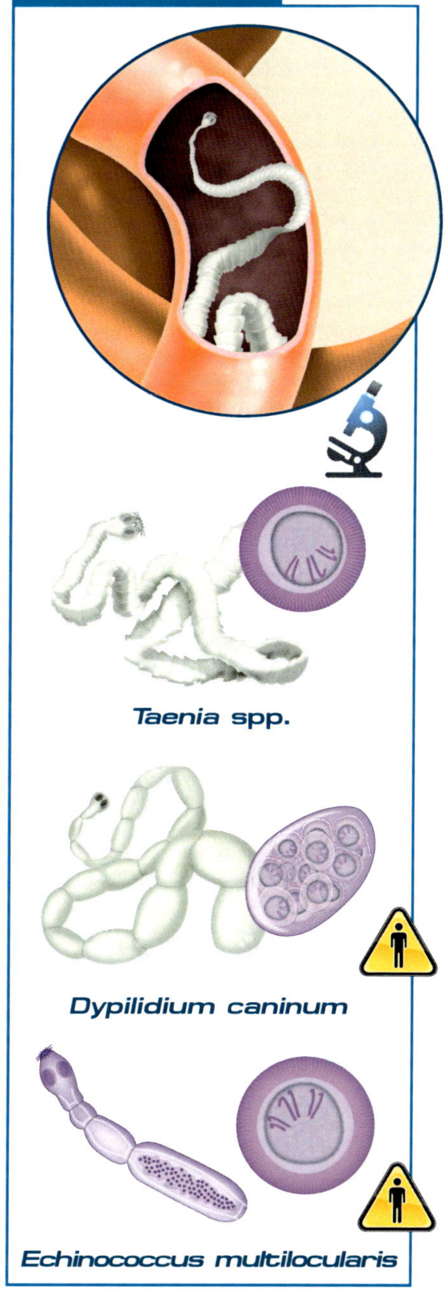

DIGESTIVE SYSTEM

46 Feline gastrointestinal inflammatory disease

Group of gastrointestinal disorders characterised by inflammation of the digestive mucosa. Multifactorial origin: genetic and immune alterations and alterations of the digestive bacterial flora.

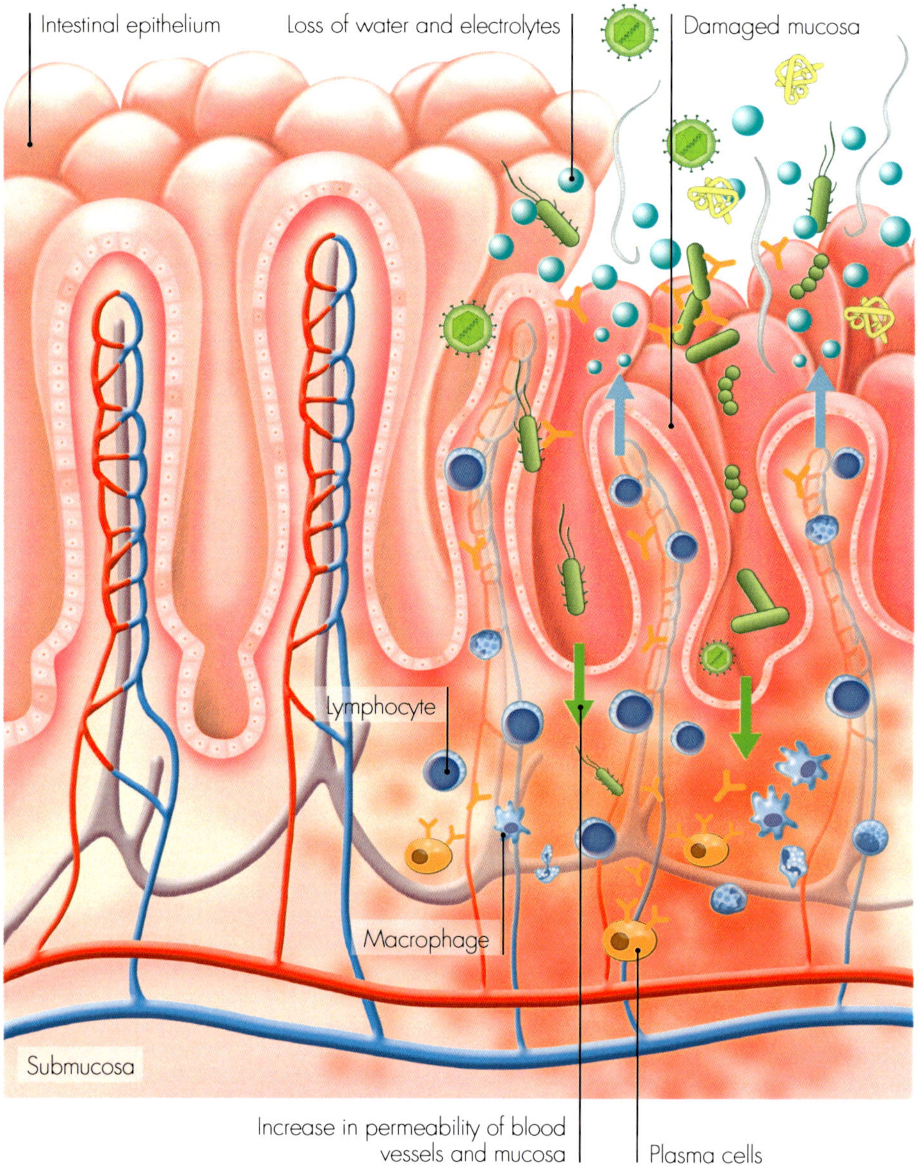

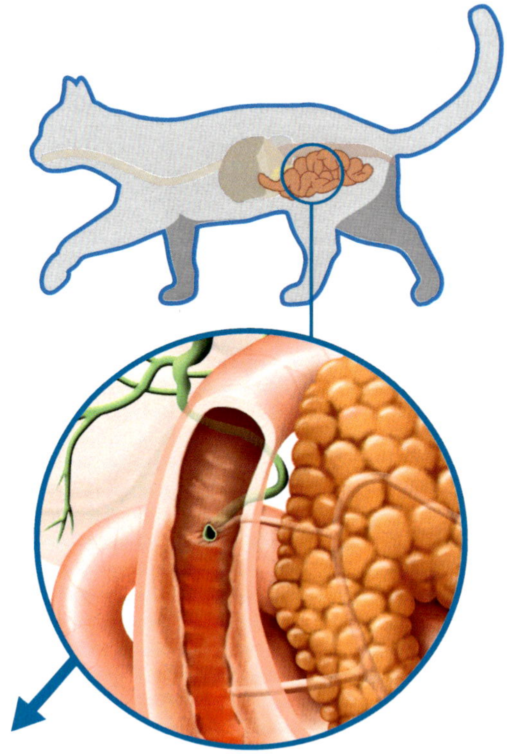

Clinical signs

- Chronic gastrointestinal signs (more than 3 weeks) with variable severity (periods of improvement and periods of relapse): vomiting, diarrhoea, anorexia, loss of weight, disorders of the appetite.
- No response to dietary modifications or symptomatic treatments.

It is the disease most frequently diagnosed in cats with vomiting and/or chronic diarrhoea.

Medical treatment

- Corticosteroids.
- Metronidazole.
- Treatment with more potent immunosuppressors is not usually necessary.

Dietary treatment

Hypoallergenic diet (novel or hydrolysate).

Diagnosis

- Rule out other causes of intestinal inflammation: parasites, endocrinopathies, adverse reaction to food, etc.
- Biopsy.

DIGESTIVE SYSTEM

47 Toxoplasmosis

Disease caused by the protozoan *Toxoplasma gondii*. In cats (definitive hosts), the parasite goes through an enteroepithelial cycle. Oocysts are released in the faeces and become infective in the exterior environment. The severity of the clinical picture depends on the affected organ, on the degree of necrosis (cell death) and on the type of strain of *Toxoplasma gondii*.

The fresh faeces of a sick cat do not represent a risk of infection. A 24-hour to 5-day period must pass for them to be infectious.

Disease transmissible to humans (zoonosis).

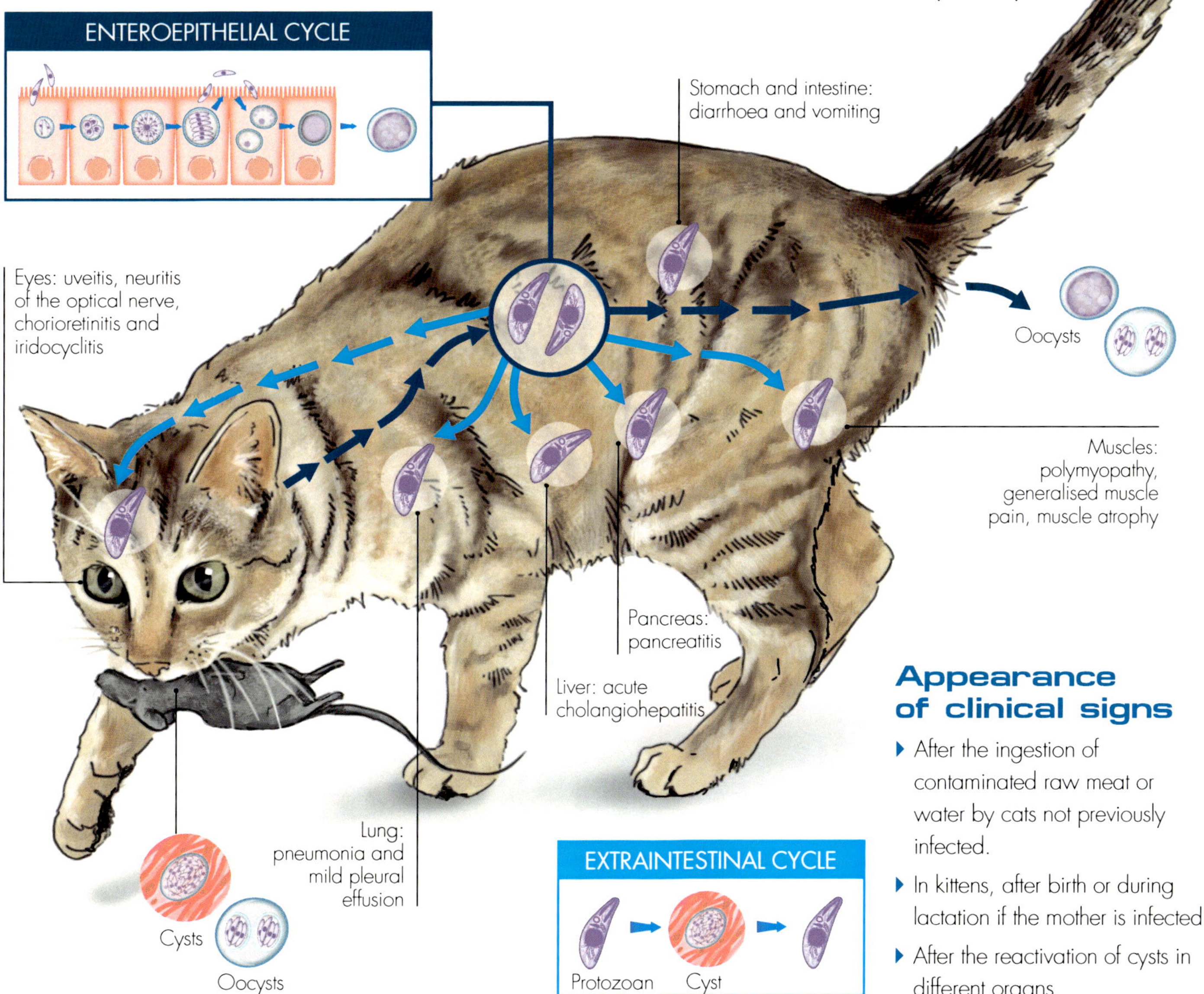

Appearance of clinical signs

- After the ingestion of contaminated raw meat or water by cats not previously infected.
- In kittens, after birth or during lactation if the mother is infected.
- After the reactivation of cysts in different organs.

Recommendations

To avoid infection, pregnant women and other people should:

- Eat meat cooked at high temperatures.
- Eat rare-cooked meat only if it has previously been frozen for two days.
- Wash their hands after gardening or cooking.
- Not drink untreated water.
- Clean the cat's litter trays daily, using a shovel and washing hands afterwards.

DIGESTIVE SYSTEM

48 Hepatic lipidosis

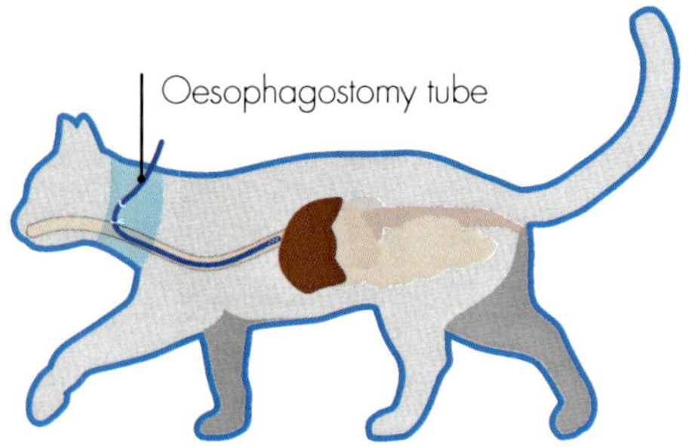

It is the accumulation of lipids in the cytoplasm of hepatocytes, which leads to improper functioning of the liver. It is the most frequent hepatic disease in cats.

Normal liver

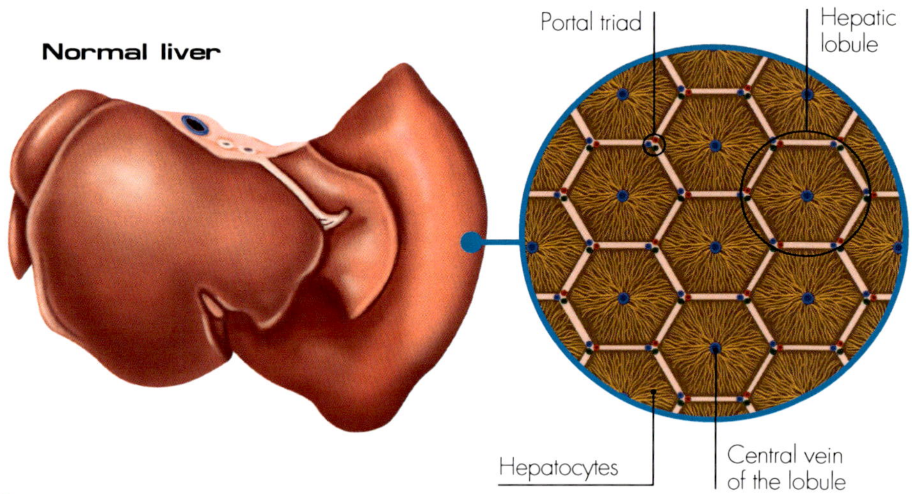

Most cats affected by hepatic lipidosis are obese before becoming sick.

Fatty liver

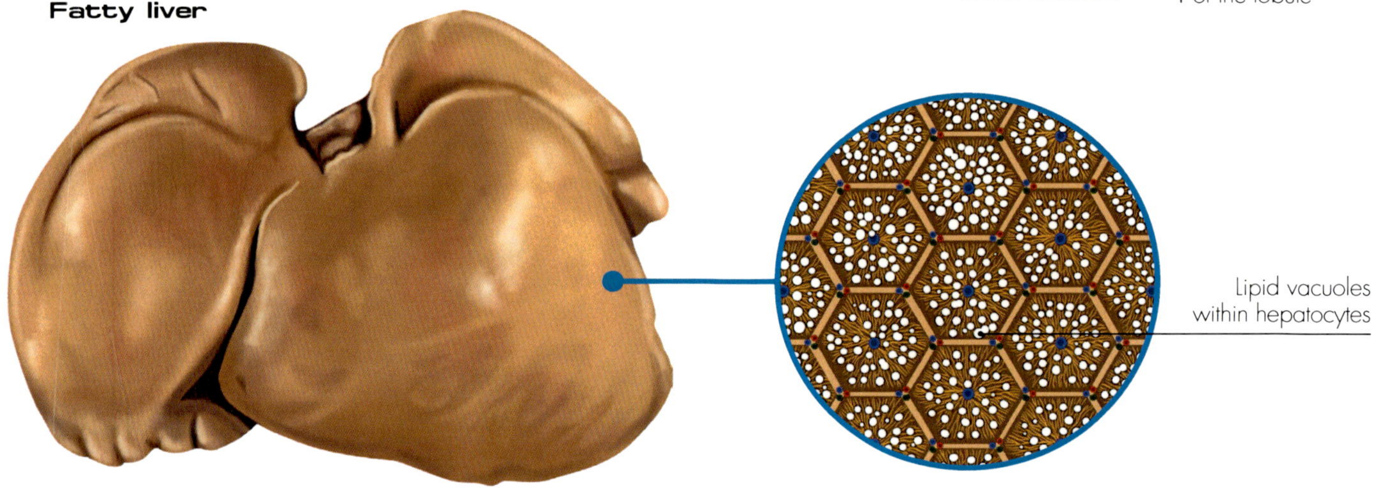

Causes

- It commonly occurs during periods of anorexia related to any disease, but also due to a smaller food intake (stress, changes in the diet, etc.).
- Lipidosis occurs in a primary form or may be secondary to another disease such as cholangiohepatitis, chronic intestinal inflammatory disease and acute or chronic pancreatitis.

Clinical signs

- Jaundice (yellowish pigmentation of the sclerae, mucosae and soft palate), anorexia and depression with intermittent vomiting.
- Other clinical signs such as ascites (free abdominal fluid) and fever are less frequent.

Medical treatment

Although the disease may be fatal, more than 60 % of cats recover with intensive nutritional therapy by means of an oesophagostomy tube and medical treatment.

DIGESTIVE SYSTEM

49 Cholangitis

Cholangitis is an inflammation of the bile ducts. There are two forms of cholangitis: the neutrophilic form, which is caused by the passage of bacteria from the intestine to the biliary tract, and the lymphocytic form, due to an immune-mediated process.

Bacteria can also spread from the intestine to the pancreas and liver by haematogenous route.

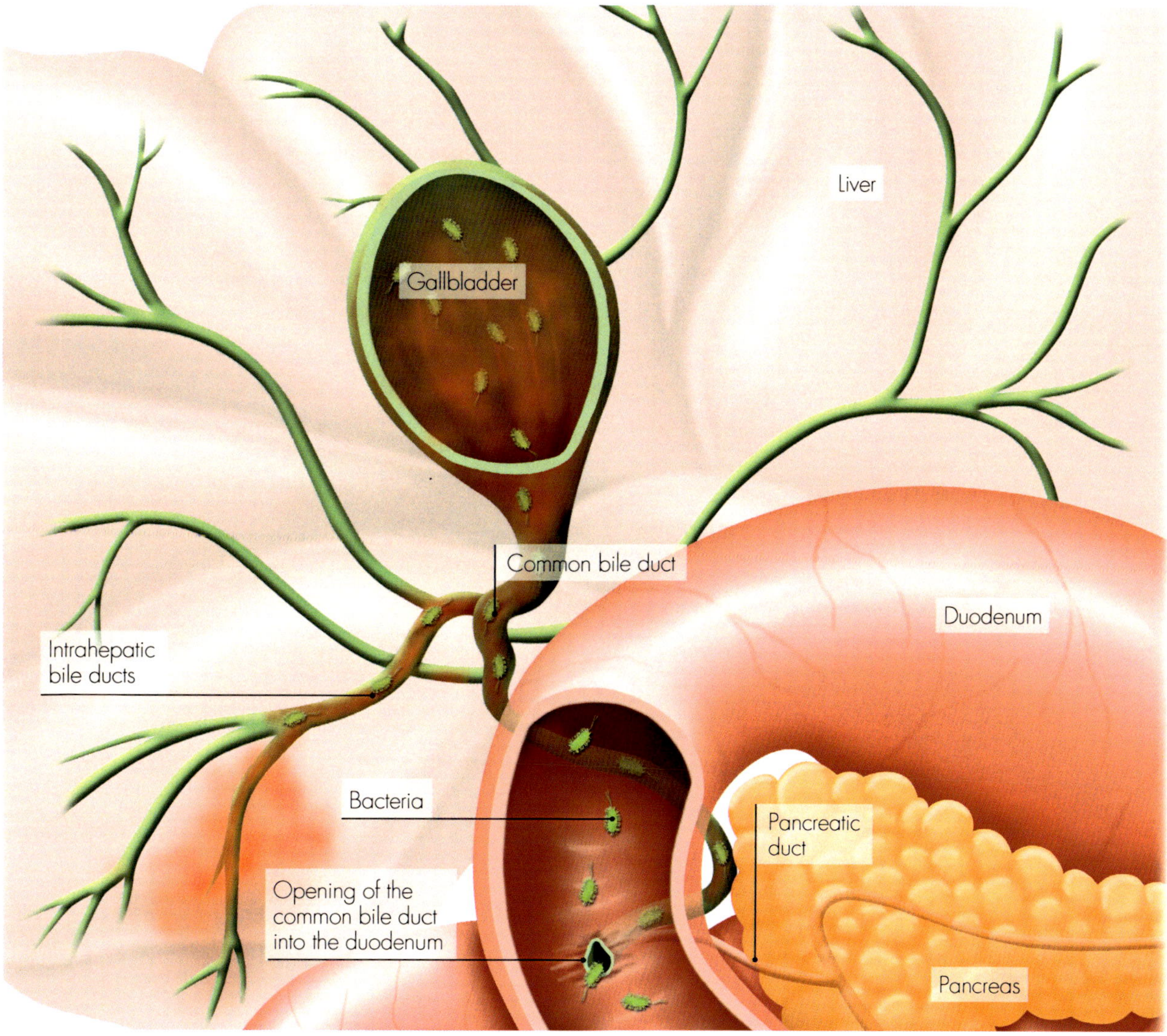

Clinical signs

- Anorexia and lack of energy.
- Loss of weight.
- Fever in the case of neutrophilic cholangitis.
- Jaundice.
- Hepatomegaly.
- Free abdominal fluid, especially in cases of lymphocytic cholangitis.

Diagnosis

It requires multiple tests to differentiate both conditions:

- Blood analysis (liver function).
- Abdominal ultrasound scan.
- Bile culture.
- Collection of biopsies (ultrasound-guided or by means of laparoscopy or laparotomy).
- Abdominal surgery in case of biliary obstruction.

DIGESTIVE SYSTEM

50 Pancreatitis and triaditis

Triaditis is the concurrence of pancreatitis, intestinal inflammatory process and cholangitis. It occurs because, in cats, the pancreatic duct joins the common bile duct before opening into the duodenum.

On some occasions, infectious agents, bile or pancreatic secretions may pass from one organ to another through this common duct, originating triaditis.

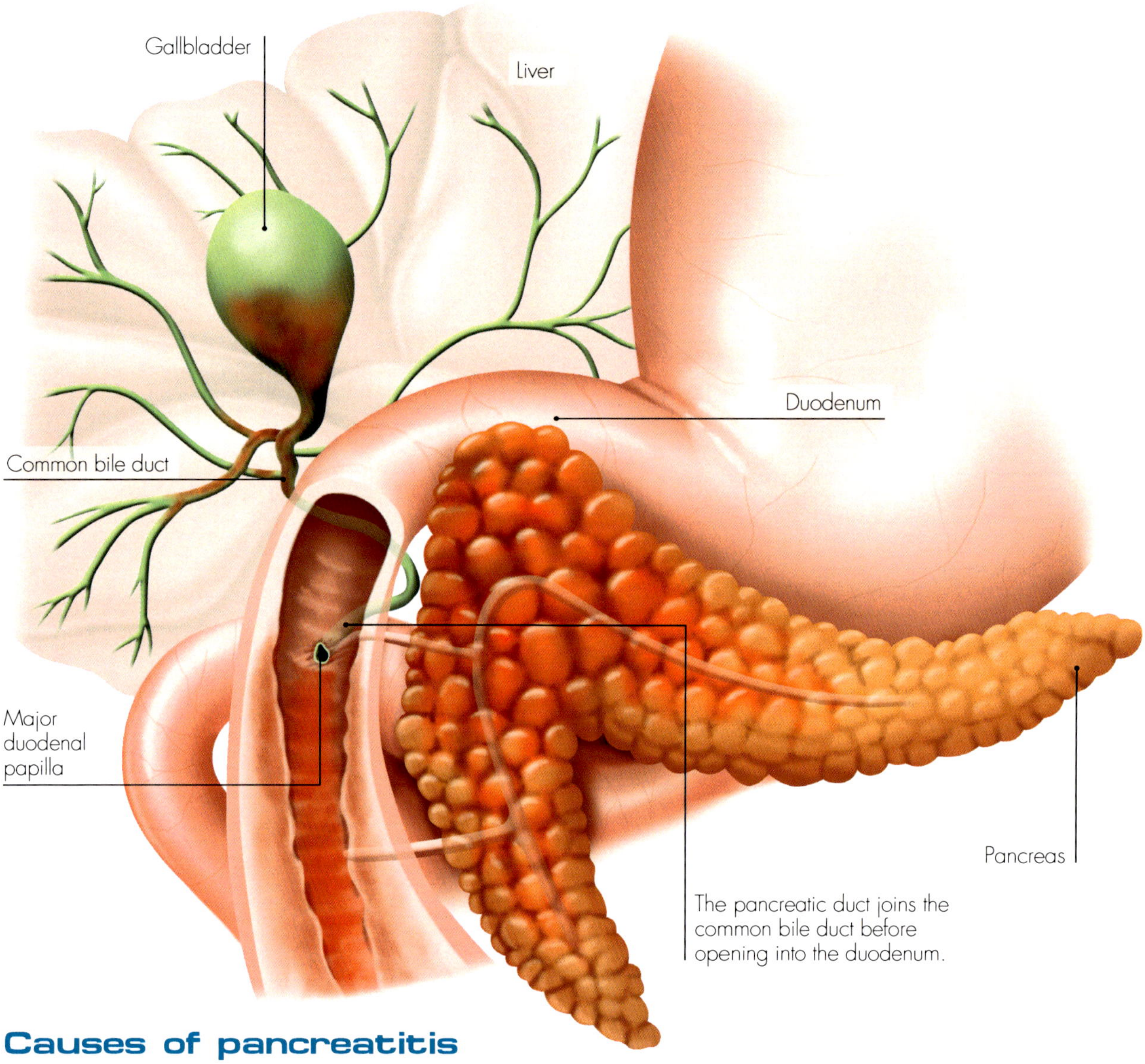

Causes of pancreatitis

- Drugs and toxic substances (organophosphates)
- Infectious agents: *Toxoplasma gondii*, hypervirulent calicivirus, FIP virus, panleukopaenia virus, herpesvirus.
- Trauma.
- Hypotension.
- Obstruction due to neoplasm.
- Duodenal reflux caused by intestinal inflammatory reflux.
- Biliary reflux caused by cholangitis.

Clinical signs

- Very variable.
- Depression, chronic vomiting and loss of weight are the most frequent signs.
- Other: diarrhoea, dehydration, jaundice, and in severe cases dyspnoea, abdominal pain and shock.

DIGESTIVE SYSTEM

51 Intestinal obstruction due to trichobezoars

Hairballs

Trichobezoars form along the gastrointestinal tract of cats as they ingest hair while grooming.
They occur both in long-haired and short-haired cats, and are usually eliminated by regurgitation, vomiting or through faeces.

The frequent elimination of trichobezoars used to be considered normal, while this is in fact wrong.

Sign of disease

The frequent elimination of trichobezoars, especially in short-haired cats, is a sign of:

- Cutaneous problem: increased grooming (external parasites, hypersensitivity, etc.).
- Inflammatory digestive problem: gastrointestinal inflammatory disease, adverse reaction to food, etc.

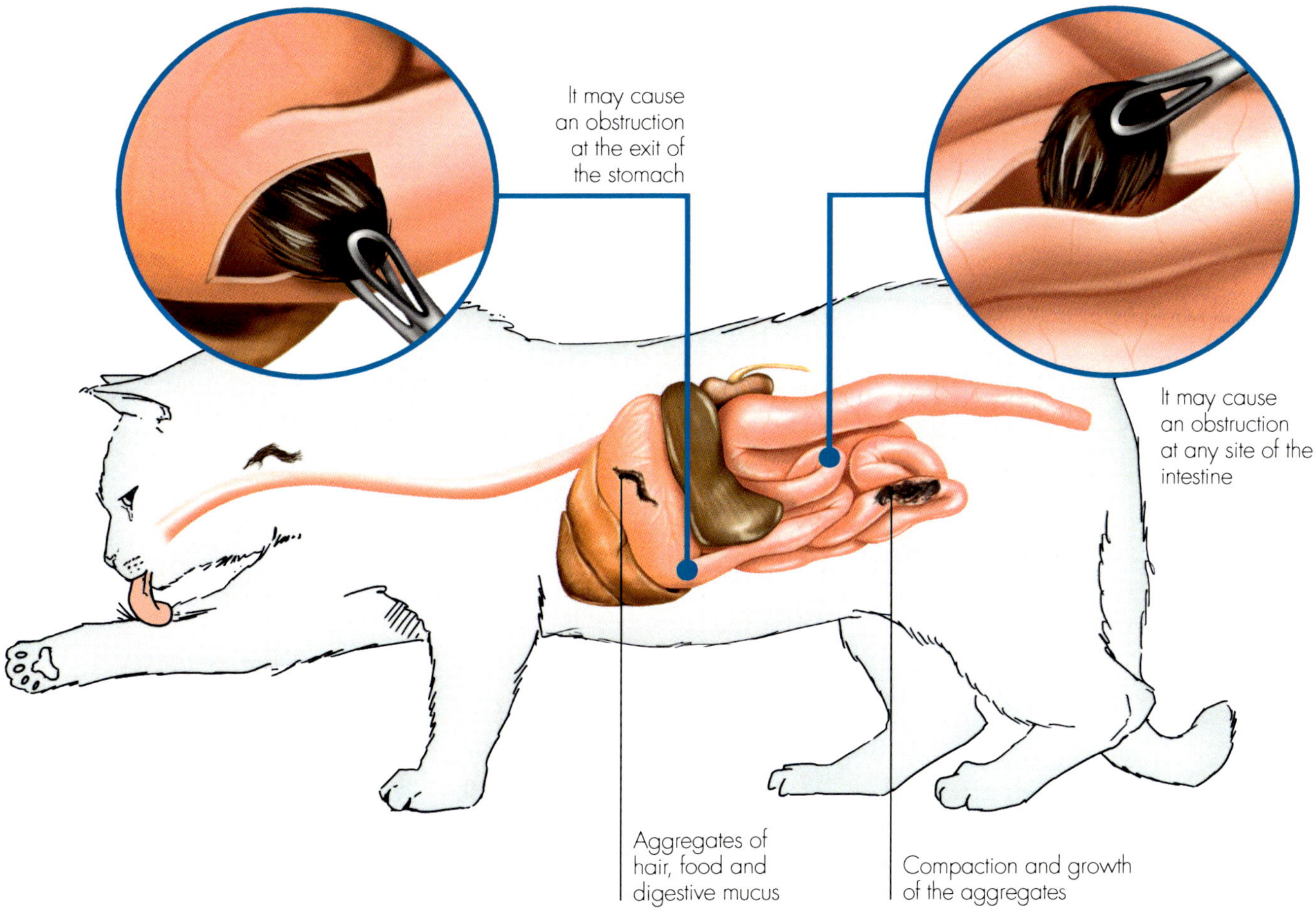

Surgical treatment

Severe obstruction: removal by means of surgery or endoscopy.

Recommendations:

- Diagnosis of digestive or dermatological diseases.
- Frequent brushing, especially in long-haired breeds and during the shedding season.
- Administration of multiple small amounts of food to facilitate gastric emptying.
- Fibre-rich diets or specific diets to reduce the formation of trichobezoars.

DIGESTIVE SYSTEM

52 Megacolon

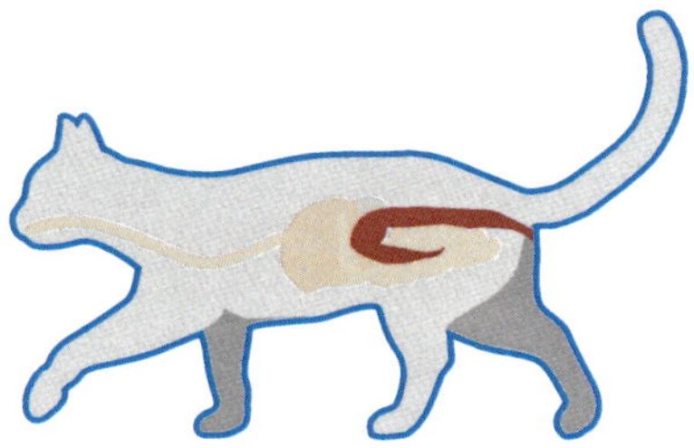

Megacolon is defined as a dilation of the large intestine. A functional anomaly of the colon causes faecal material to accumulate and prevents its elimination.

If the maximum diameter of the colon/the length of L5 > 1.6 on the radiograph → diagnosis of megacolon.

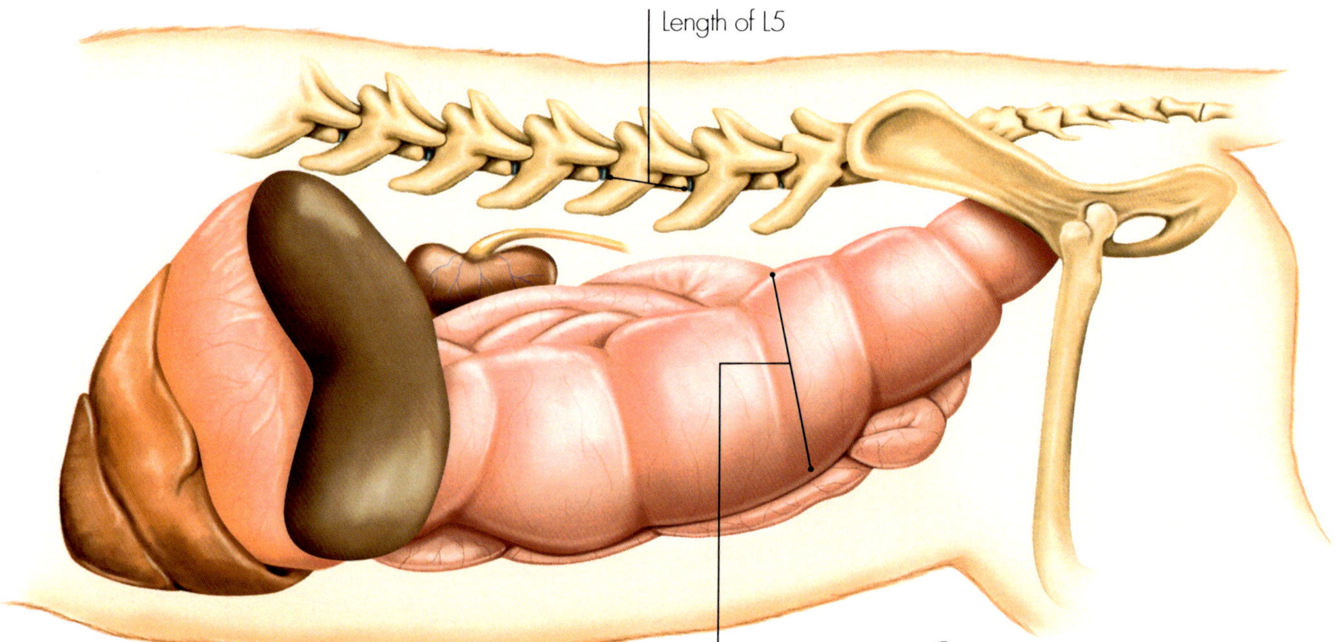

⚠ The diagnosis requires abdominal and hip radiographs as well as a neurological examination.

Classification

- **Congenital:** due to problems in the development of some of the segments caused by anatomical abnormalities or neurological development problems.
- **Secondary to an obstruction:** due to stenosis, masses, neoplasms, etc.
- **Idiopathic megacolon:** generally in cats from 8 years old. Dysfunction of the smooth muscle of the colon leading to severe chronic constipation and subsequently megacolon.

Clinical signs

- Chronic constipation.
- Tenesmus: painful and unproductive attempts to defecate (meows).
- Faeces out of the litter tray (aversion due to pain).
- Bloody fluid similar to diarrhoea (irritation of the mucosa).
- Vomiting in severe clinical pictures, due to irritation of the colon and absorption of toxins.
- Anorexia, lethargy and weakness.

Medical treatment

- Enemas in cases of severe constipation.
- Laxatives by oral route.
- Prokinetic drugs such as ranitidine.

Surgical treatment

- Applied if the drug therapy is not effective.
- Subtotal colectomy is the technique of choice, 85-95 % of the colon is removed.

Dietary treatment

Diets rich in insoluble fibres.

NERVOUS SYSTEM

53 Central, peripheral and autonomic nervous system

Central nervous system

1. Brain
2. Cerebellum
3. Spinal cord
4. Brainstem
5. 5th lumbar vertebra
6. 6th lumbar vertebra
7. Spinal cord
8. Cauda equina

Peripheral nervous system

9. Cervical spinal nerves
10. Brachial plexus (C5, C6, C7, T1)
11. Radial n.
12. Musculocutaneous n.
13. Median n.
14. Ulnar n.
15. Thoracic spinal nerves
16. Lumbar spinal nerves
17. Lumbar plexus (L5, L6, L7, S1, S2)
18. Femoral n.
19. Saphenous n.
20. Obturator n.
21. Ischial n.

Autonomic nervous system

22. Cranial cervical ganglion
23. Distal vagal ganglion
24. Vagosympathetic trunk
25. Caudal cervical ganglion
26. Cervicothoracic ganglion
27. Vagus n.
28. Vagus n., dorsal branch
29. Vagus n., ventral branch
30. Ganglia of the sympathetic trunk
31. Celiac-mesenteric ganglion
32. Caudal mesenteric ganglion
33. Hypogastric n.

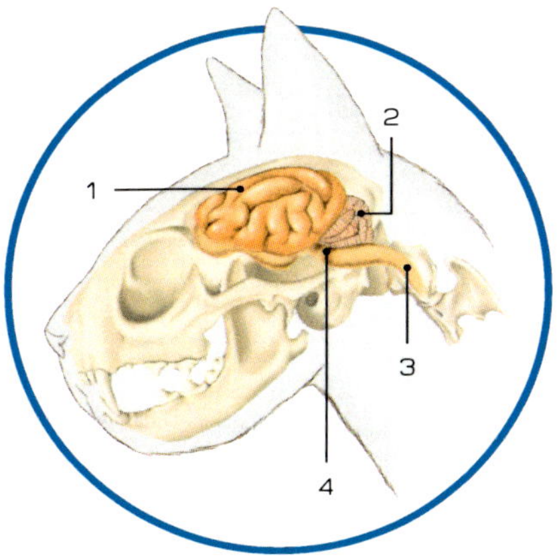

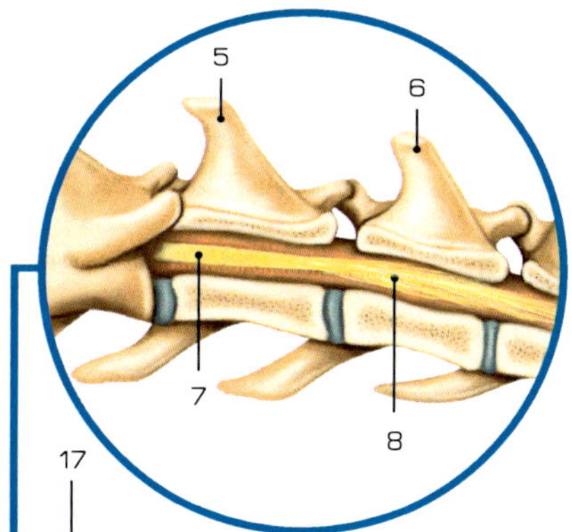

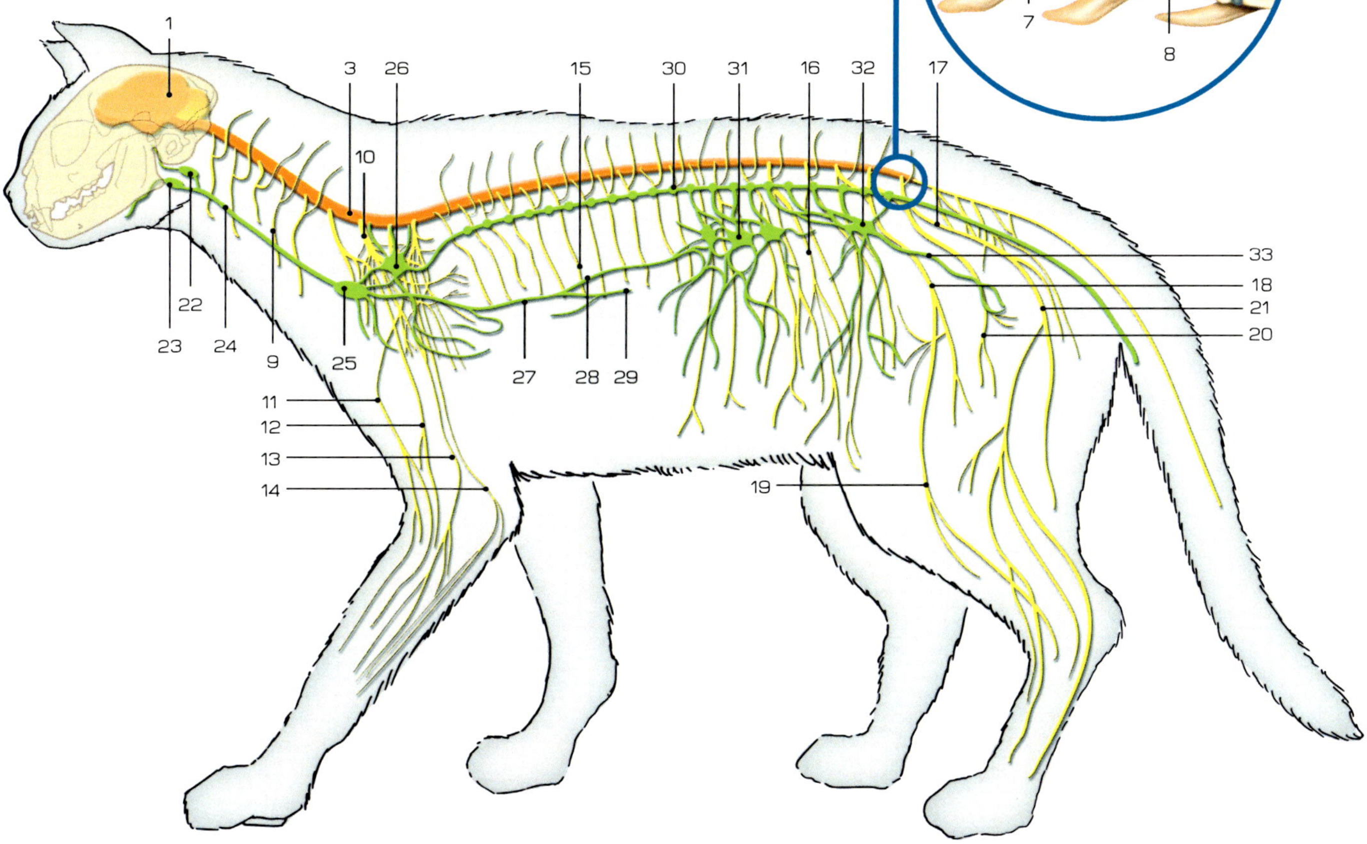

EYES

54 Structures of the eye

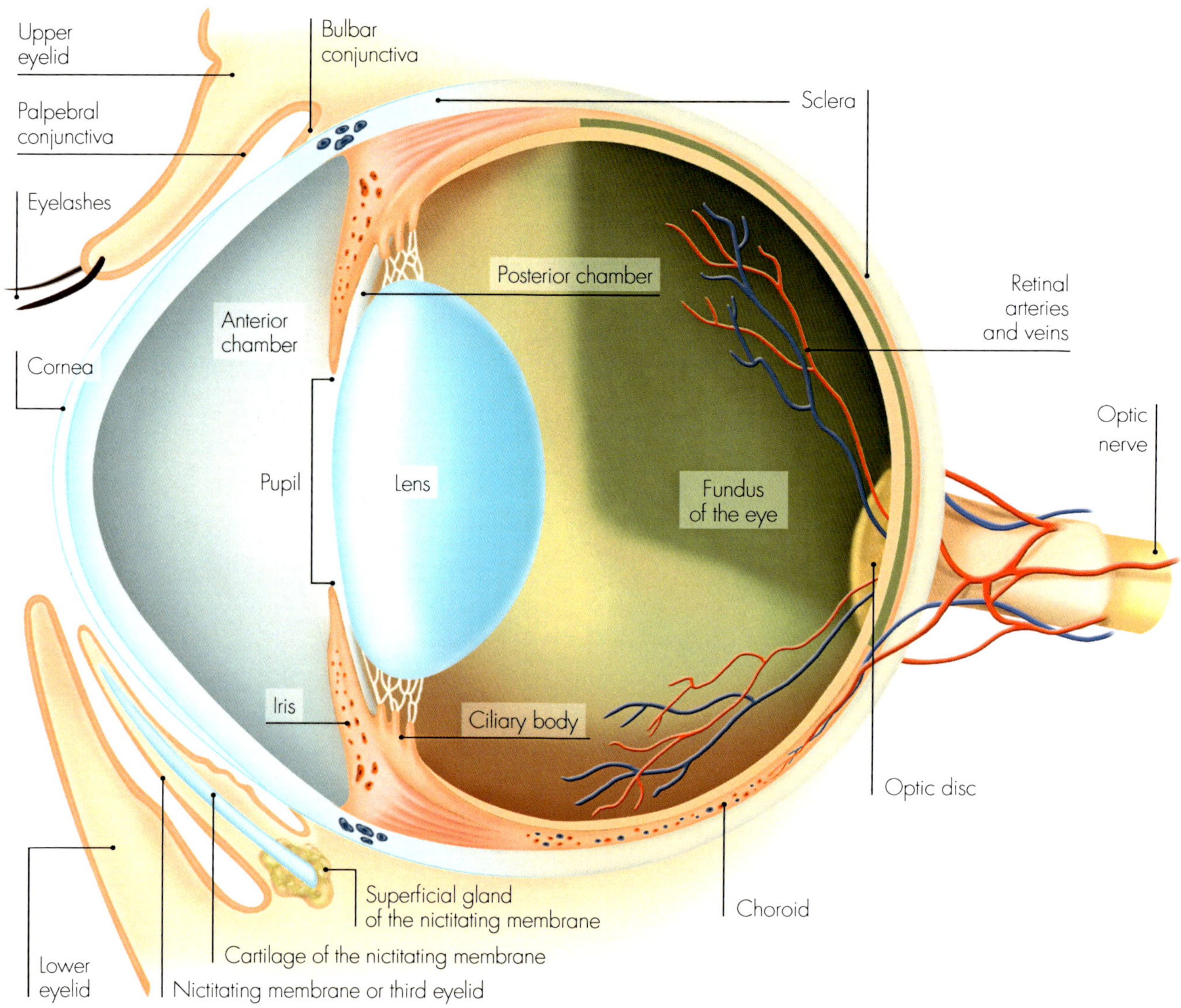

Mechanism of pupillary reflex

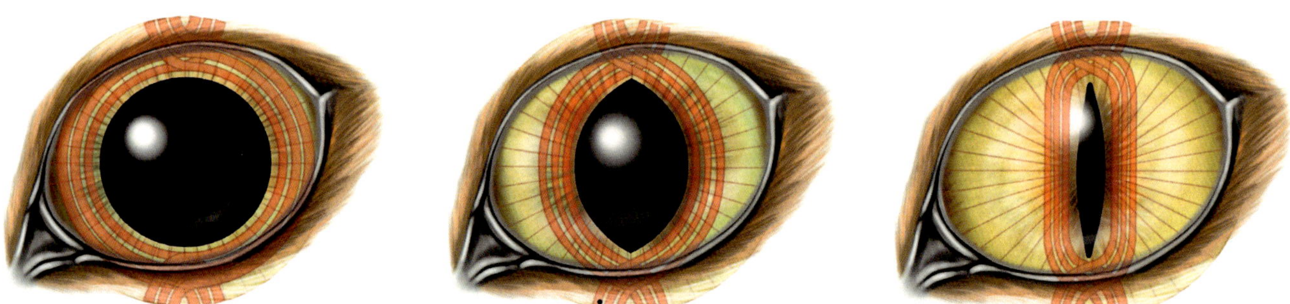

EYES

55 Corneal ulcer and keratitis

Surgical treatment of severe ulcers

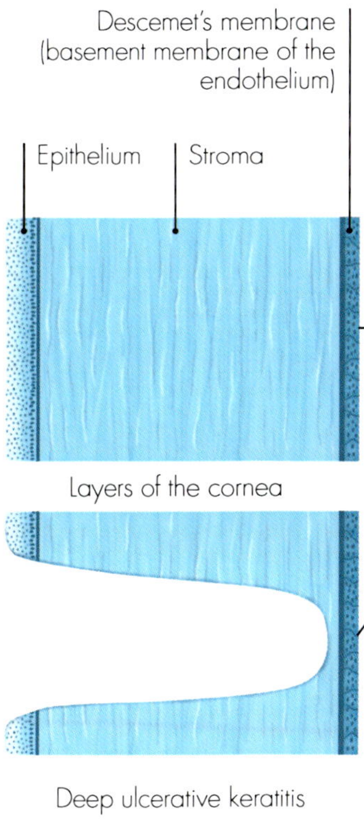

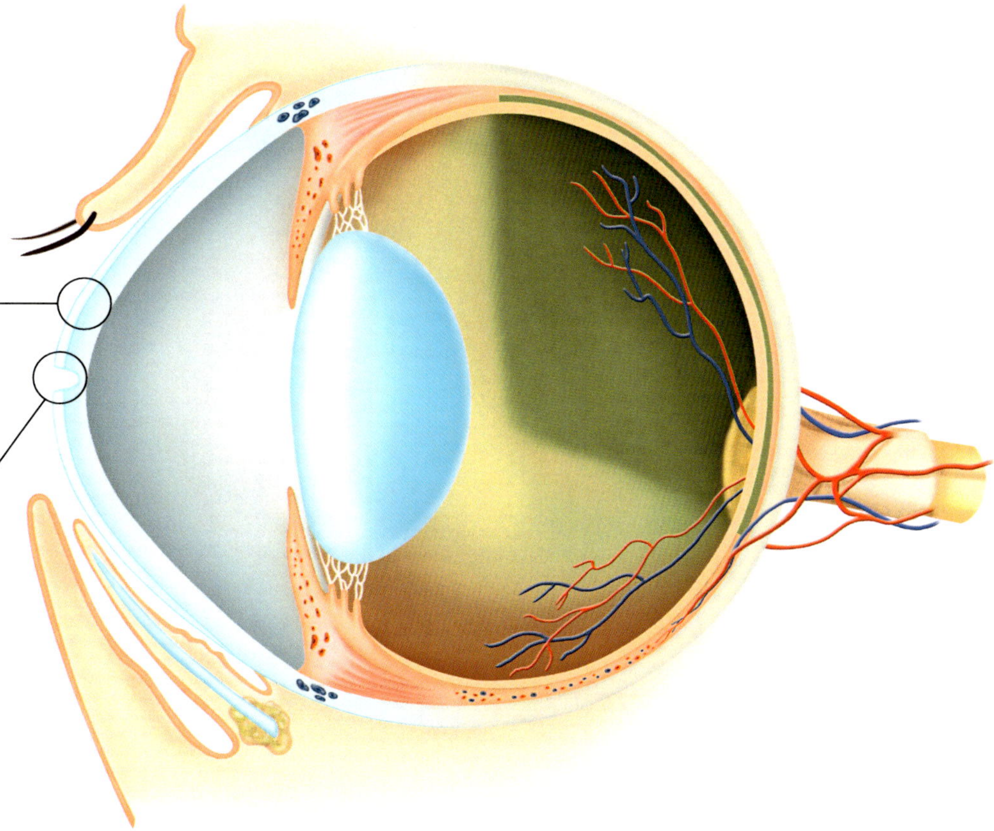

Surgery of deep ulcerative keratitis by means of a conjunctival flap

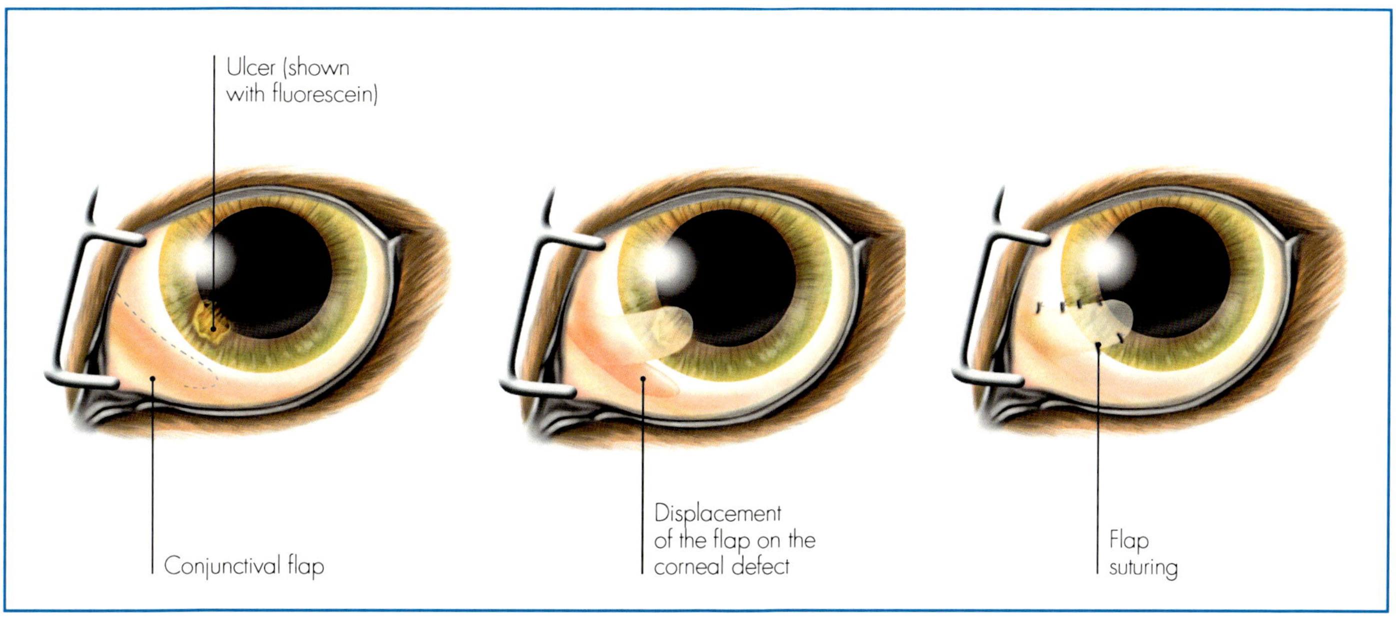

56 Feline infectious peritonitis (FIP)

The mutation of the feline coronavirus (FCoV) turns it into the FIP virus. The infection with FCoV is very common in cats all around the world, but only 5-10 % of the infected cats develop FIP. Transmission occurs through faeces.

Risk factors

- Groups of cats (shared litter tray).
- Age: cats under one year of age are the most affected.
- Stress (overcrowding, poor hygiene) and co-infections with other viruses.

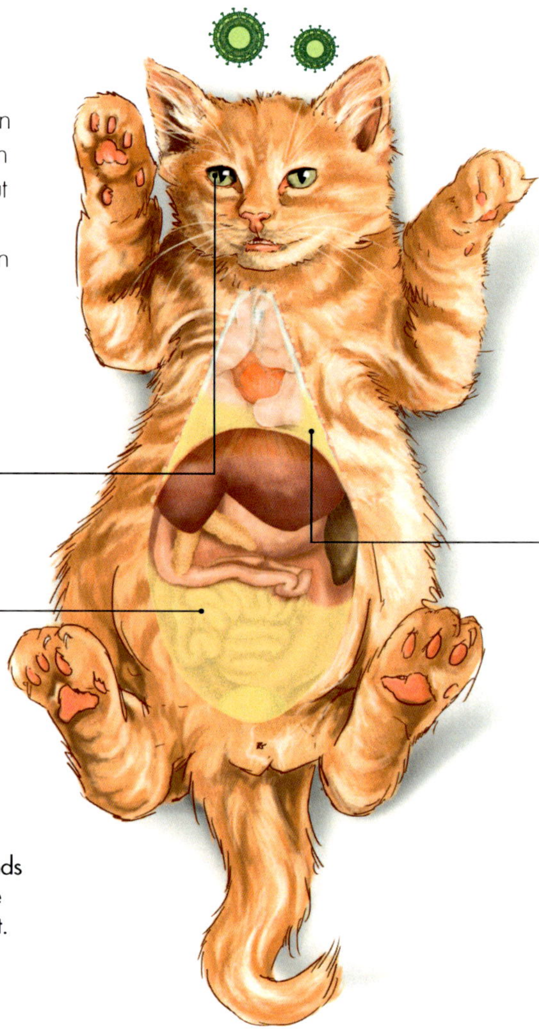

Wet form

Clinical signs

Common signs in both the dry and wet forms:

- Fever with no response to antibiotic treatment.
- Depression.
- Progressive loss of weight.
- Growth problems in kittens.

⚠ The progression of the disease depends on the interaction of the virus with the immune system of each individual cat.

Dry form

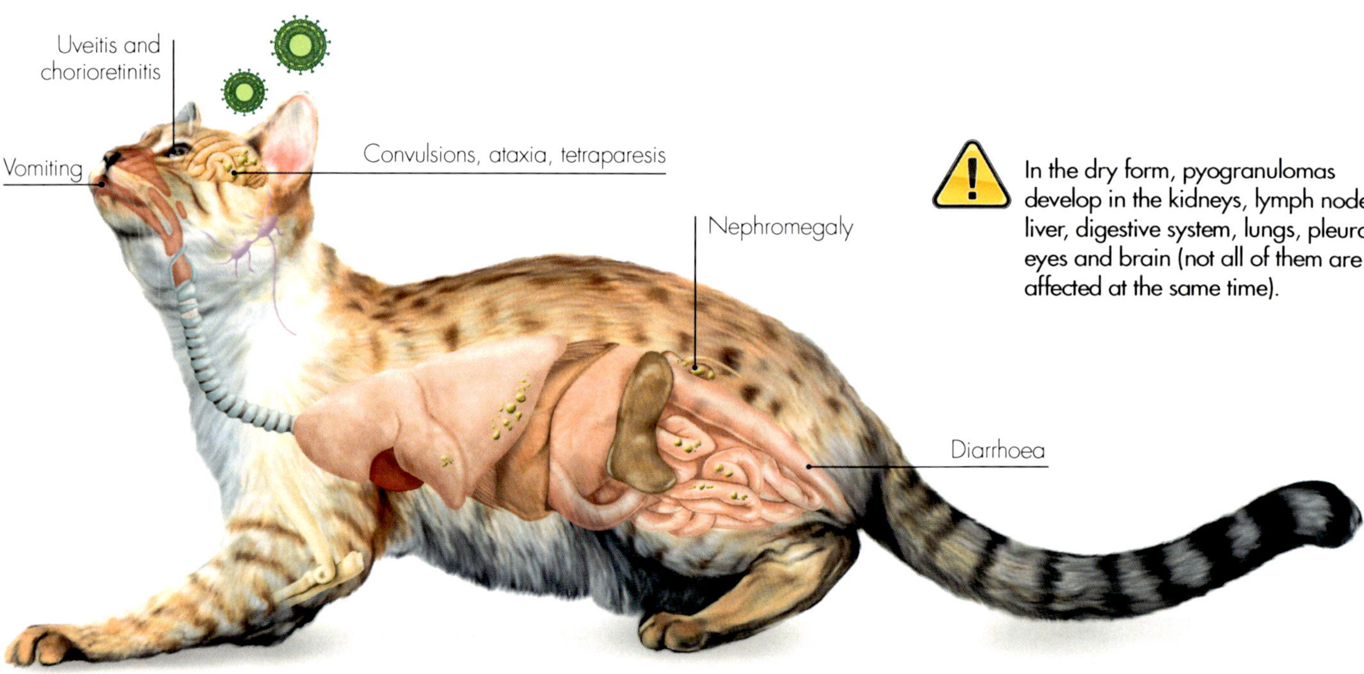

⚠ In the dry form, pyogranulomas develop in the kidneys, lymph nodes, liver, digestive system, lungs, pleura, eyes and brain (not all of them are affected at the same time).

57 Feline leukaemia (FeLV)

The feline leukaemia virus is mainly transmitted through saliva and requires close and prolonged contact between cats. On a less frequent basis, it is transmitted through nasal discharge, tears, faeces, urine, milk, semen, vaginal fluids and placenta.

The vaccine should first be administered at 8-9 weeks of age, followed by a booster injection 3-4 weeks later. After that, the cat should be vaccinated a year later and then annually when living in a risk environment.

The diagnosis of feline leukaemia is complex, and tests such as ELISA or PCR of both blood and bone marrow samples may be necessary.

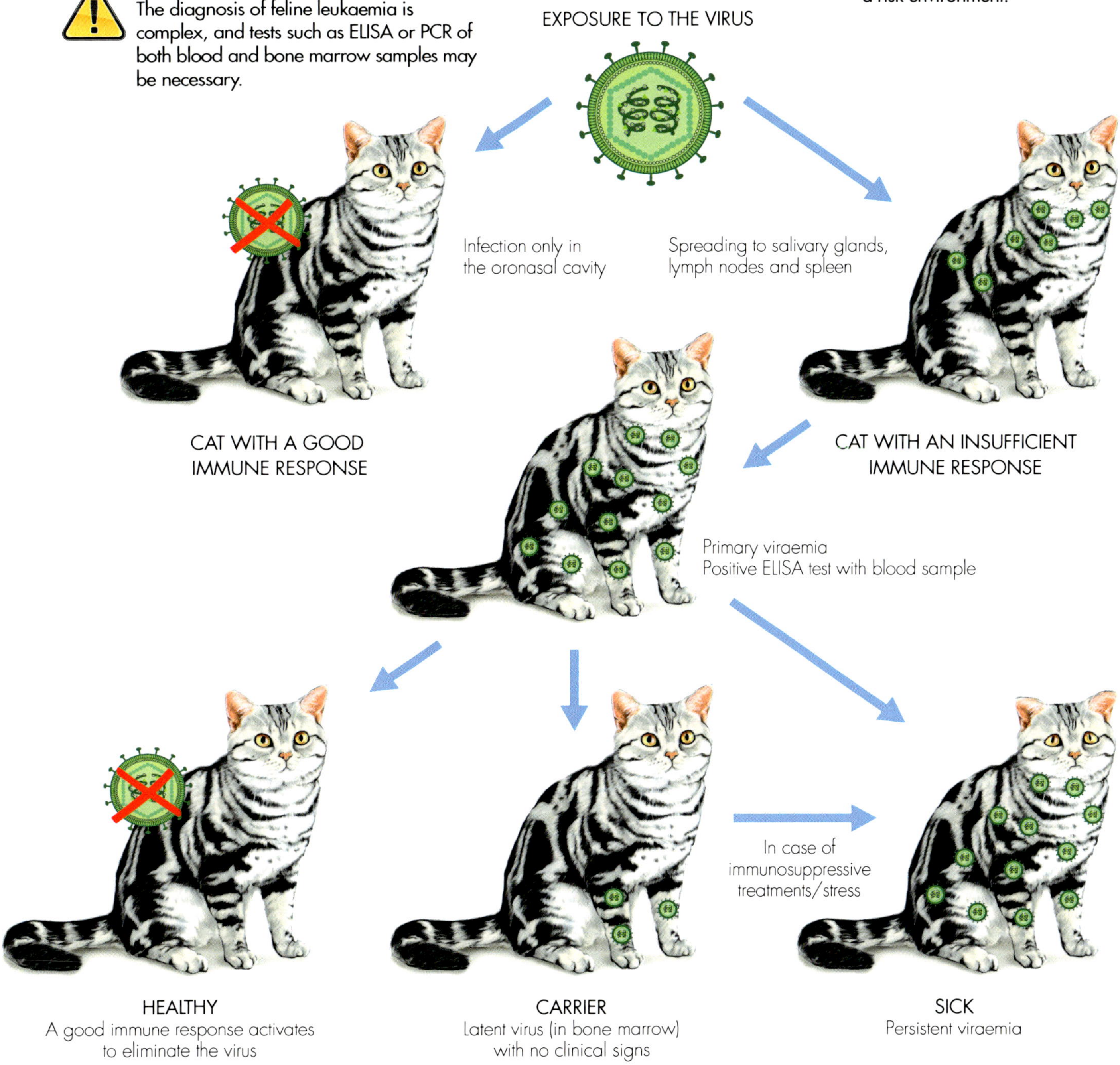

Medical treatment

There is no curative treatment available to date, but the symptoms can be relieved and life expectancy increased.

58 Feline immunodeficiency (FIV)

This viral infection is essentially transmitted through saliva or blood in cases of bites.
An infected mother may transmit it to 50 % of her offspring during gestation and lactation.

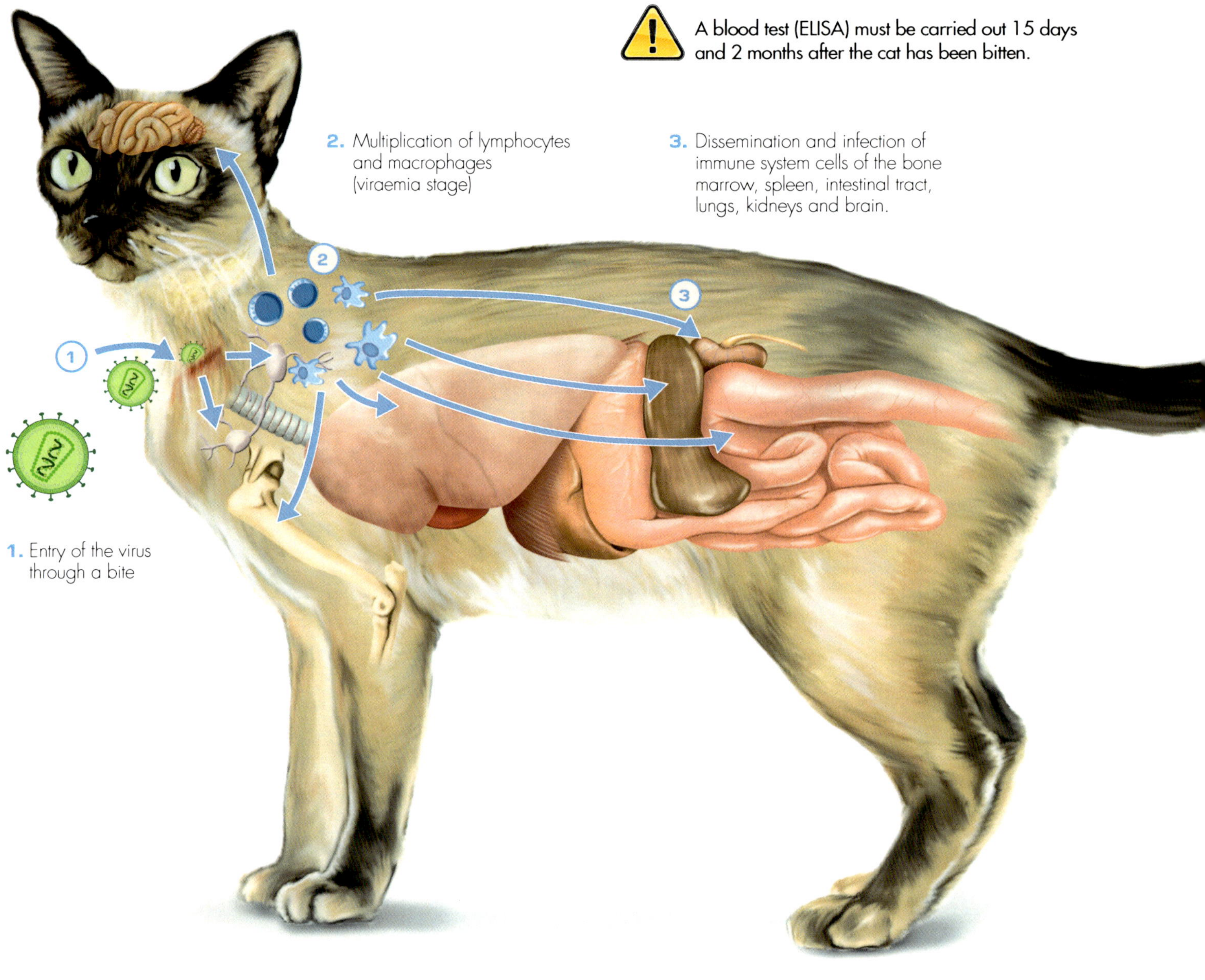

Clinical signs

- When the infection occurs: fever, enlargement of the lymph nodes, apathy and anorexia.
- This is followed by an asymptomatic period that may last for years.
- When the immune system is weakened, an immune-deficiency stage (AIDS) that lasts for several months appears: fever, anorexia, lymph node enlargement, secondary infections (diarrhoea, otitis, conjunctivitis, rhinitis, cutaneous abscesses), gingivostomatitis, immune-mediated anaemia, neurological disorders and tumours.

Diagnosis

- Detection of antibodies in blood in cats > 6 months (ELISA) and PCR in cats < 6 months.
- Any positive result should be confirmed by a PCR test.

59 Feline panleukopaenia

Disease caused by a parvovirus. Some variants of canine parvoviruses may affect cats. Infection occurs through direct contact with secretions of a sick cat (faeces, saliva, etc.) or with a contaminated environment.

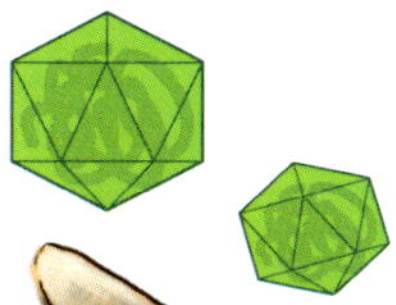

⚠ Its infective capacity is very high, since it survives on any surface for up to a year and is resistant to most disinfectants. It causes death in a high percentage of non-vaccinated and insufficiently vaccinated cats.

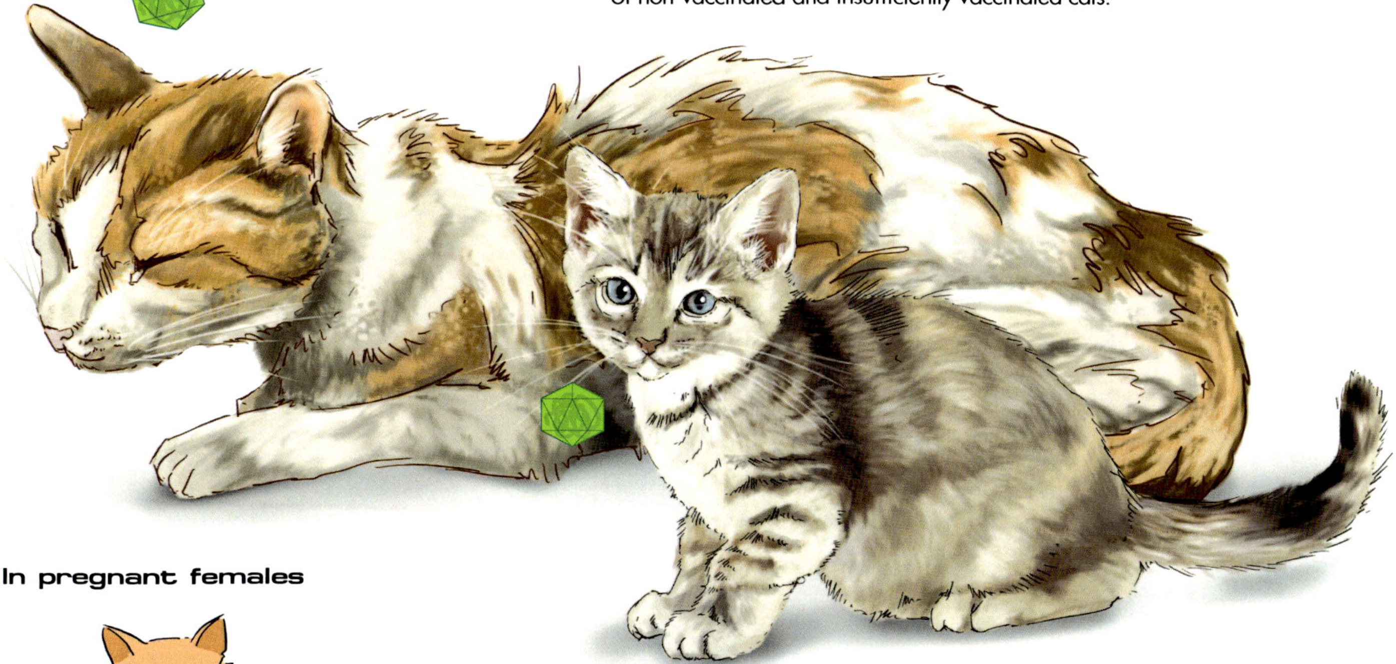

In pregnant females

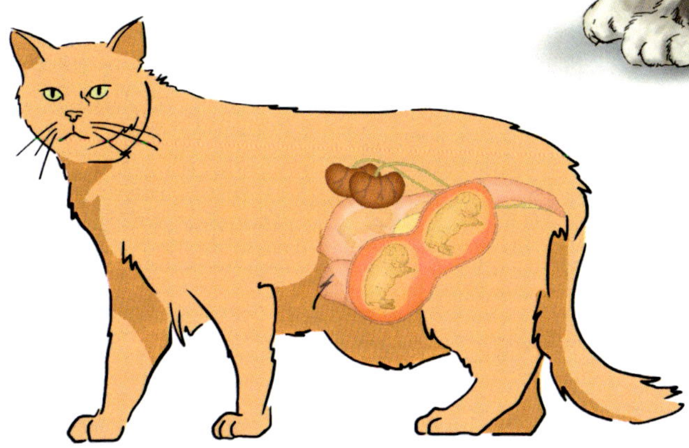

GESTATION (2 MONTHS)		
Early infection	Mid-gestation infection	Late infection
Foetal death and resorption	Abortions and foetal mummification	Birth of kittens with lesions in the brain and cerebellum

Clinical signs

They occur between 5 and 14 days after exposure to the virus:

- Fever, intense depression.
- Anorexia, vomiting.
- Sepsis with haemorrhagic diarrhoea and jaundice.
- Sudden death in cats of up to 1 year of age.

Recommendations

- Disinfect all the areas in contact with the sick cat with bleach diluted at 1:30 for 10 minutes.
- Only correctly vaccinated cats should enter the areas that could not be appropriately cleaned.

⚠ All the cats should be vaccinated, even indoor cats due to the risk of infection through shoes, clothes, etc.

60 Feline rhinotracheitis

Herpesvirus

Type I feline herpesvirus is the causative agent of feline rhinotracheitis. It is transmitted through direct contact with nasal, ocular and pharyngeal secretions of sick cats. It can also be transmitted through our hands and contaminated objects, although in a less effective manner.

It is one of the main agents responsible for the feline respiratory disease complex, together with calicivirus, *Bordetella bronchiseptica*, *Chlamydophila felis* and *Mycoplasma* spp.

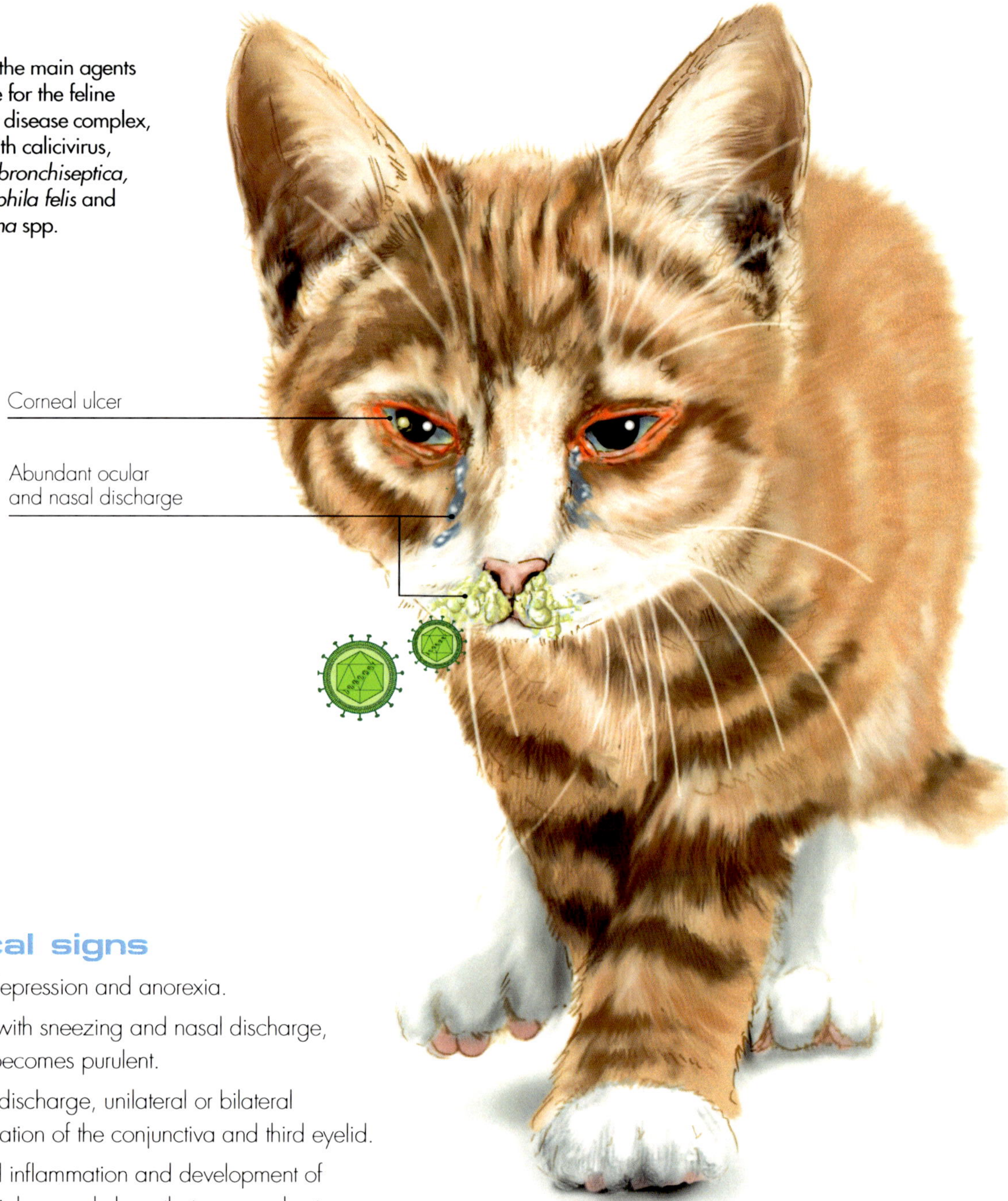

Clinical signs

- Fever, depression and anorexia.
- Rhinitis with sneezing and nasal discharge, which becomes purulent.
- Ocular discharge, unilateral or bilateral inflammation of the conjunctiva and third eyelid.
- Corneal inflammation and development of superficial corneal ulcers that may evolve to deep corneal ulcers and even corneal sequestra.
- Uncommon: ulcers in the mouth, hypersalivation, cough and facial ulcers.

Almost 80 % of cats infected by the herpesvirus become carriers for the rest of their lives. Stress and immunosuppressive treatments may reactivate it.

61 Feline calicivirus

It is a very infectious virus that is widespread among cats. It can be transmitted through saliva, tears, nasal secretions, faeces and urine of sick animals or chronic carriers of the virus. Our hands and objects are another source of infection.

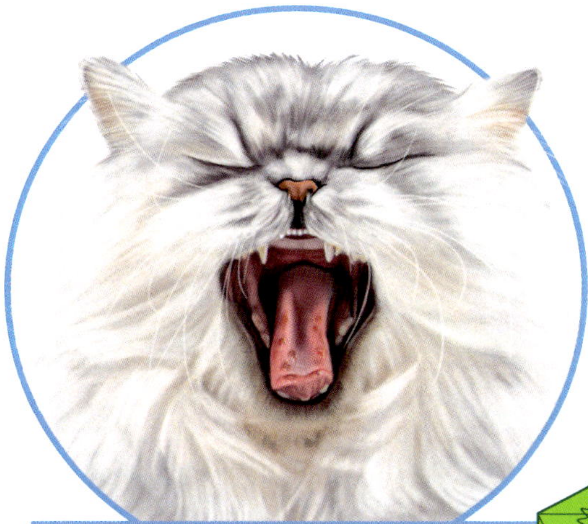

Oral ulcers and nasal discharge

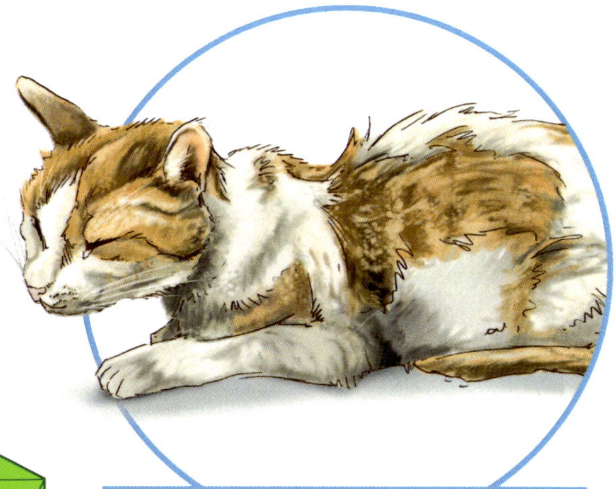

Virulent systemic calicivirus

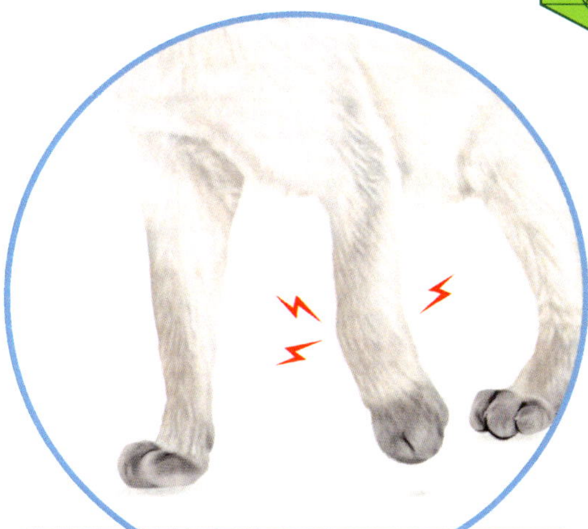

Lameness (polyarthritis)

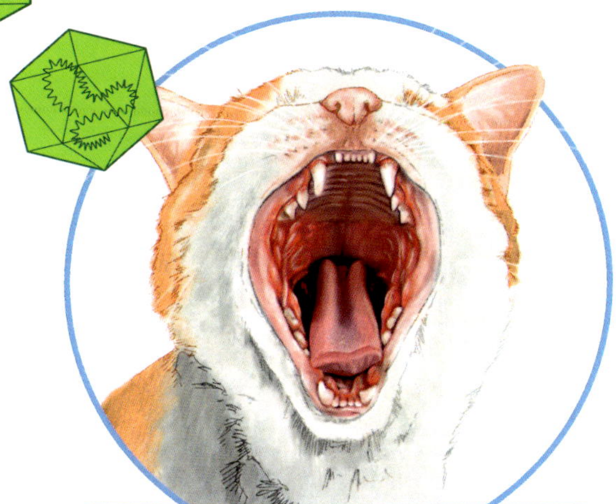

Chronic gingivostomatitis

Vaccines do not prevent the animal from being infected, but are very effective to reduce the severity of the clinical signs.

Recommendations:

- The environment can be disinfected with sodium hypochlorite (bleach) diluted at 1:32 in water.
- Hands can be disinfected with 70 % ethanol.

Clinical signs

They depend on the type of strain and its virulence:

- Acute infection:
  - Acute oral and upper airway disease, with fever, oral ulcers, sneezing and nasal discharge.
  - Virulent systemic disease: more severe in adult cats, in which it causes vasculitis.
  - Polyarthritis: transient lameness with fever.
- Chronic infection:
  - Chronic gingivostomatitis (see Chart no. 44).
  - Glomerulonephritis.

62 Feline chlamydiosis

The disease is caused by *Chlamidophyla felis* bacteria. Infection occurs through contact with conjunctival, nasal and vaginal secretions as well as through faeces. Our hands and objects (food and water bowls) may be a route of infection.

Newborn cats become infected through their mother's genital mucosa and develop severe conjunctivitis short after birth. Cats > 1 year of age run a lower risk of becoming infected as they develop immunity.

Vaccination does not completely protect against infection, but significantly reduces clinical signs. It is recommended in cats living in groups.

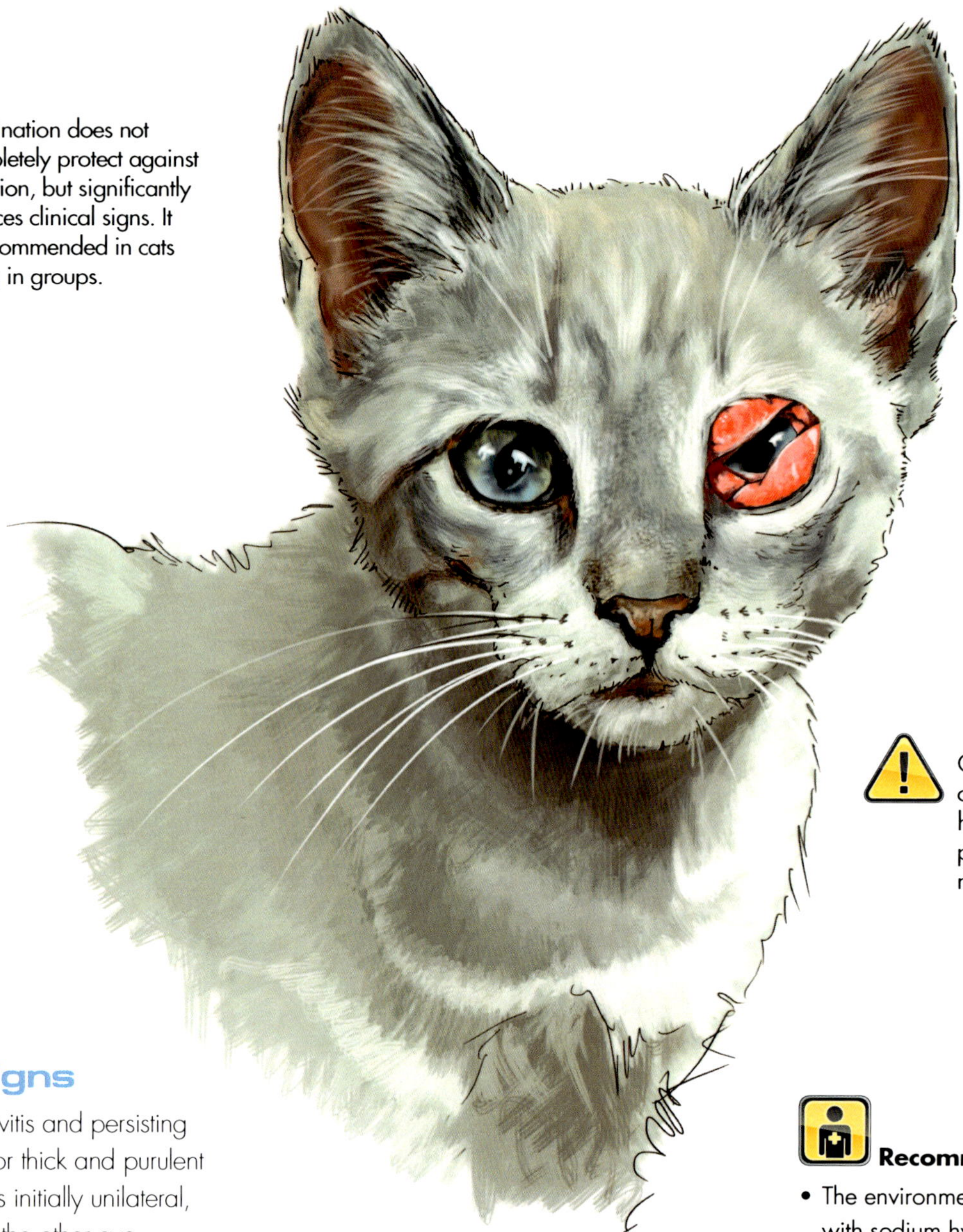

Conditions such as overcrowding, lack of hygiene, stress and poor ventilation favour reinfections.

Clinical signs

- Severe conjunctivitis and persisting tearing (watery or thick and purulent tears). Infection is initially unilateral, and then affects the other eye.
- Inflamed and half-closed eyes (blepharospasm).
- Uncommon: sneezing, nasal discharge and fever.

Recommendations

- The environment can be disinfected with sodium hypochlorite (bleach) diluted at 1:32 in water (these bacteria only survive for a few days in the environment).
- Hands can be disinfected with 70 % ethanol.

63 Bone marrow aspiration technique

Bone marrow is the most important haematopoietic organ (production of blood cells) organ in the organism.

Aspiration of bone marrow from the iliac crest

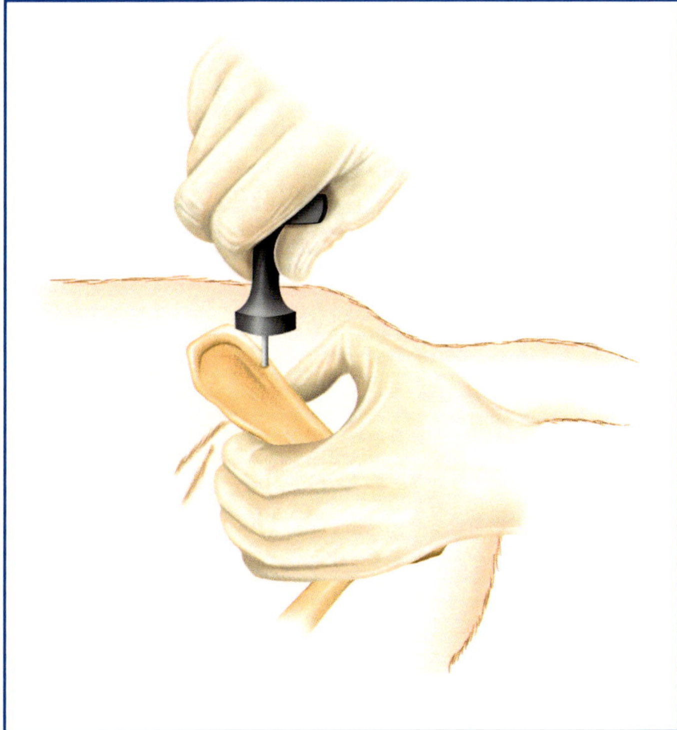

Aspiration of bone marrow from the femur

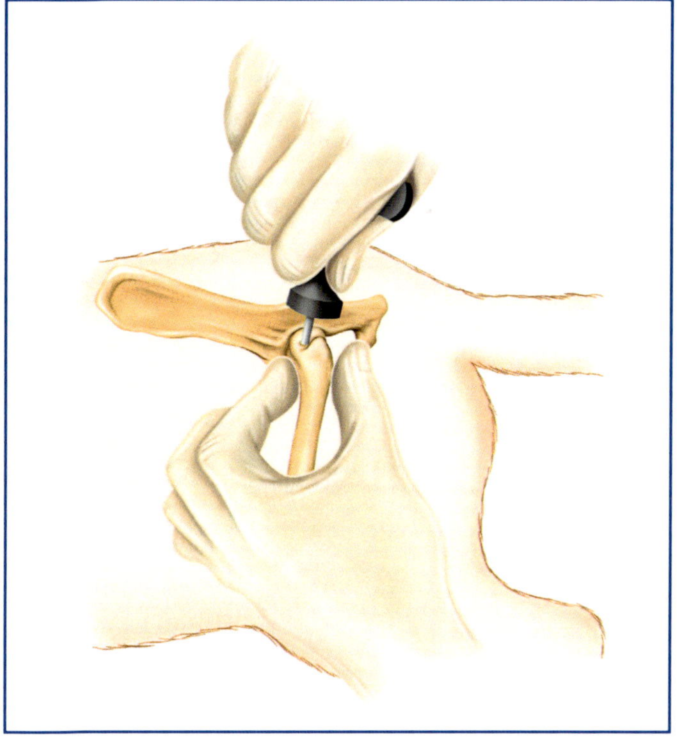

Aspiration of bone marrow from the head of the humerus

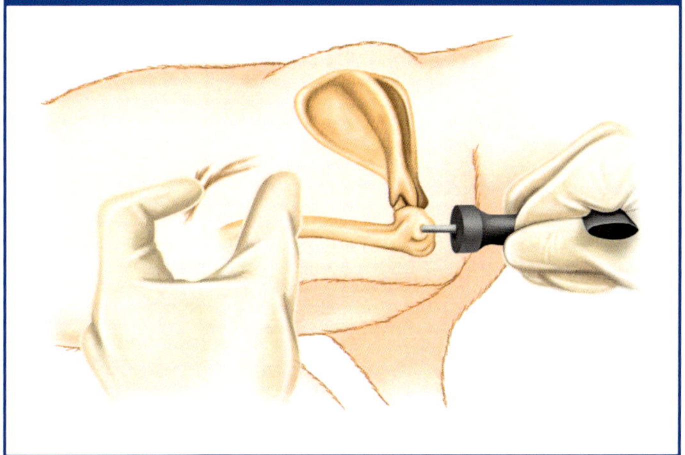

The aspiration and analysis of bone marrow is useful for the diagnosis of anaemia and infectious diseases such as feline leukaemia.

Method

- Bone marrow is aspirated by means of special needles for bone marrow, or with a hypodermal 18-gauge needle in cats with thin bones.
- The bones from which samples can be collected are the humerus, iliac crest and femur.

64 Urethral catheterisation and cystocentesis

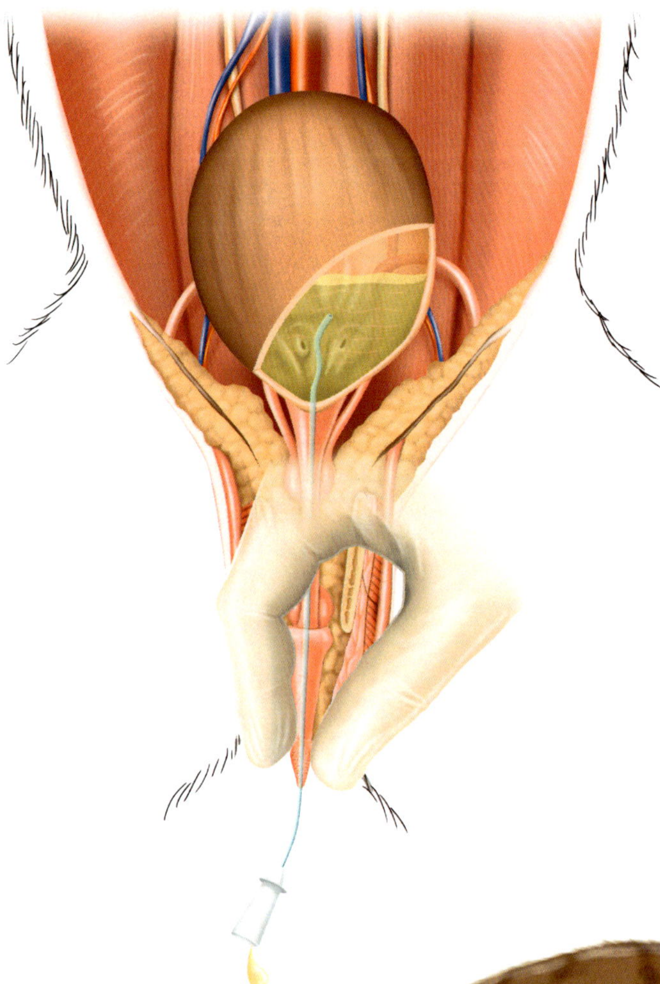

Urethral catheterisation

- It is performed in cases of urethral obstruction (the cat cannot urinate).
- It consists in introducing a catheter from the penis to the bladder, generally for a maximum of 24-48 hours.
- It always requires anaesthesia and intensive analgesic treatment.

Cystocentesis

- The collection of a urine sample by means of cystocentesis is required for the diagnosis of urine infections.
- It consists in puncturing the bladder with a thin needle.
- It is not painful.
- The urine sample obtained will be sent in a sterile container for a bacterial culture and antibiogram.

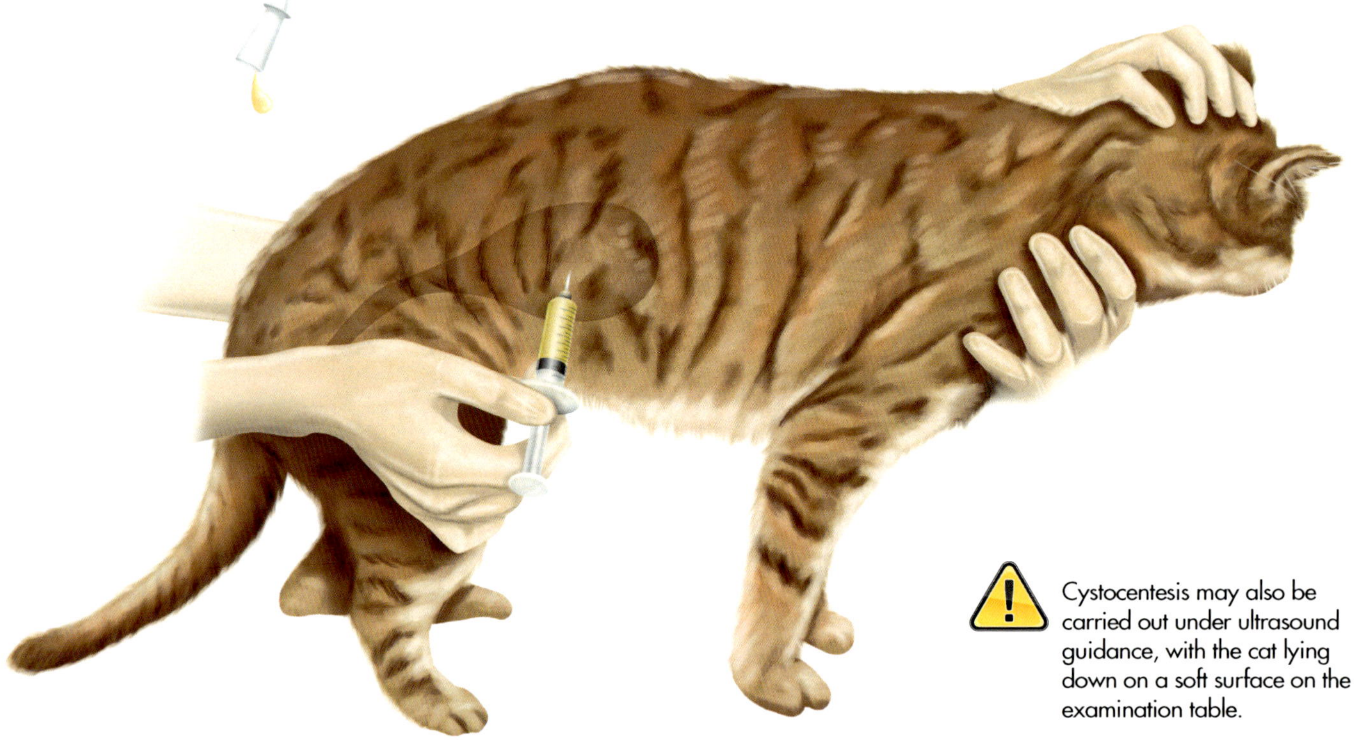

Cystocentesis may also be carried out under ultrasound guidance, with the cat lying down on a soft surface on the examination table.

65 Thoracic drainage

Thoracostomy and thoracocentesis

In cases of pyothroax, chylothorax and pneumothorax, the placement of a thoracostomy tube until the process resolver is required.

The accumulation of fluid in the pleural space causes respiratory difficulties. Its removal by means of thoracocentesis allows the diagnosis of the cause and considerably improves the patient's respiratory capacity.

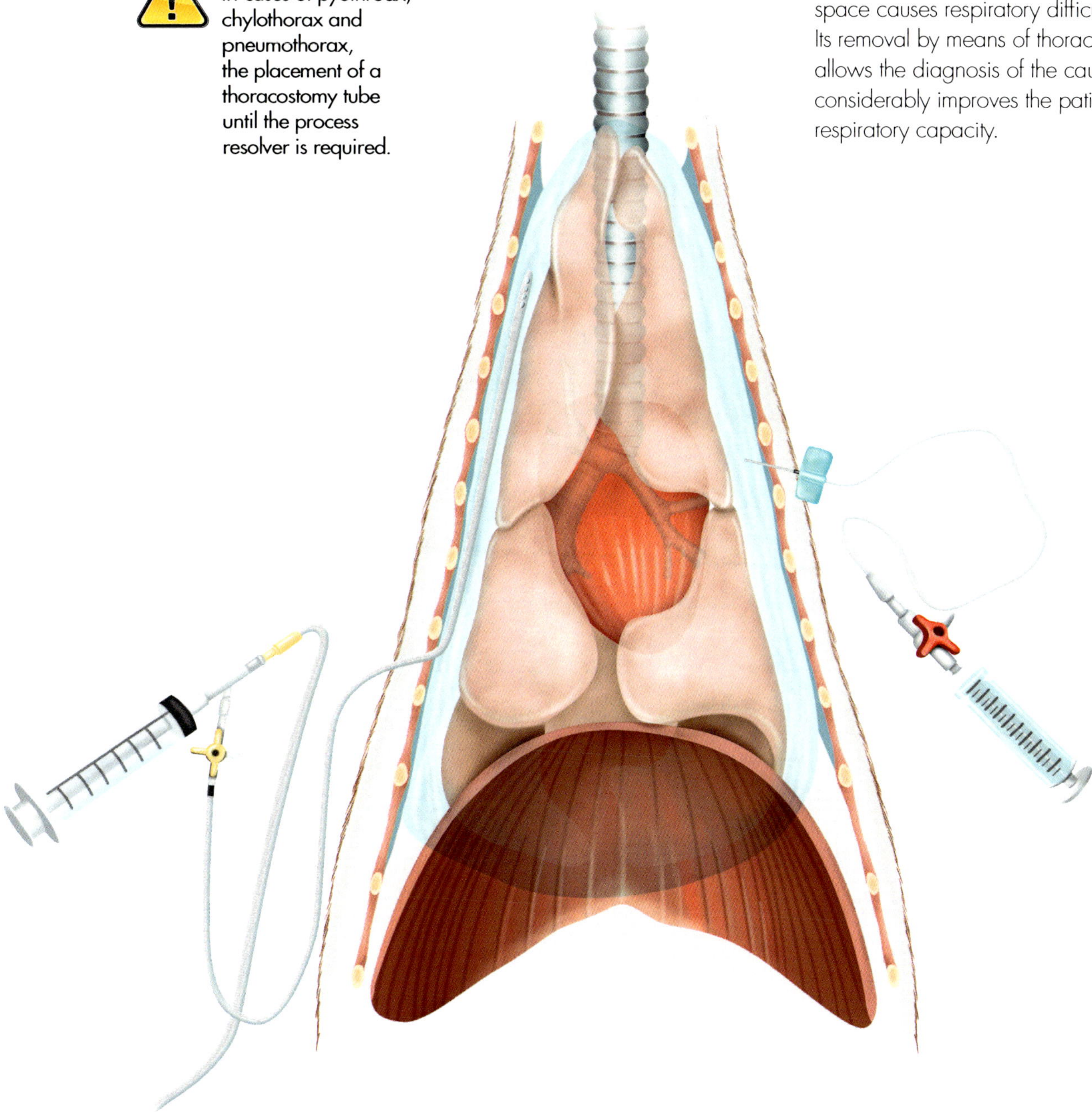

Thoracostomy with a tube

A thoracostomy consists in the placement of a thin tube into the pleural space, which allows the removal of the fluid that is continuously being formed.

Thoracocentesis

Thoracocentesis consists in the removal of accumulated pleural fluid by means of a puncture with a thin needle in the thoracic wall.

66 Feeding tubes

Feeding tube by means of oesophagostomy

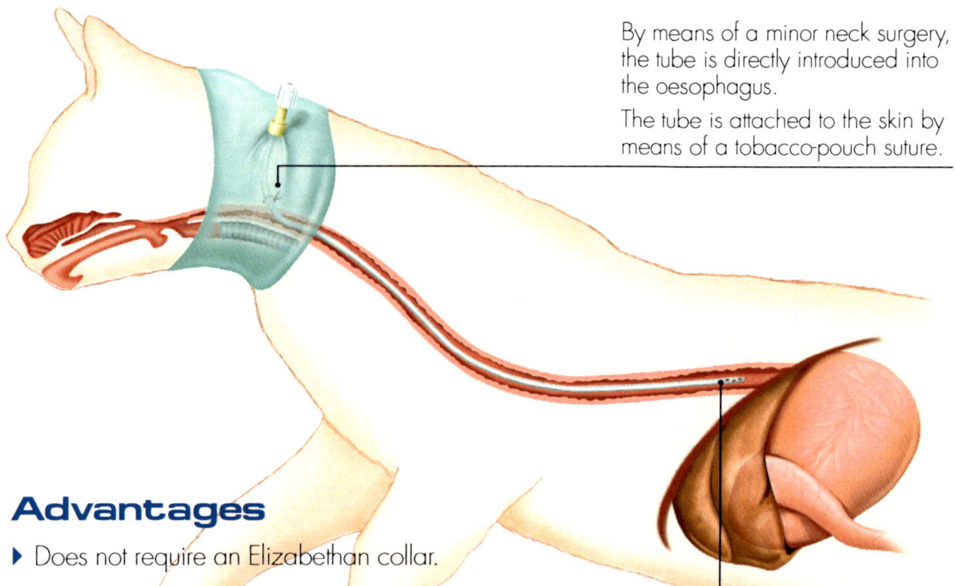

Advantages

- Does not require an Elizabethan collar.
- Does not annoy the animal.
- Can be left for up to 3 months.
- The cat can eat voluntarily at any time.
- Allows the administration of medication through the tube.

Indications

- Hepatic lipidosis.
- Anorexia caused by any disease accompanied by a loss of 20 % of the animal's weight.
- Facial trauma.
- Oral surgeries.

⚠ These systems give good results and are a better alternative to force feeding, since this latter option can lead to an aversion syndrome, which will result in the cat needing more time to eat by itself again.

Nasooesophageal tube

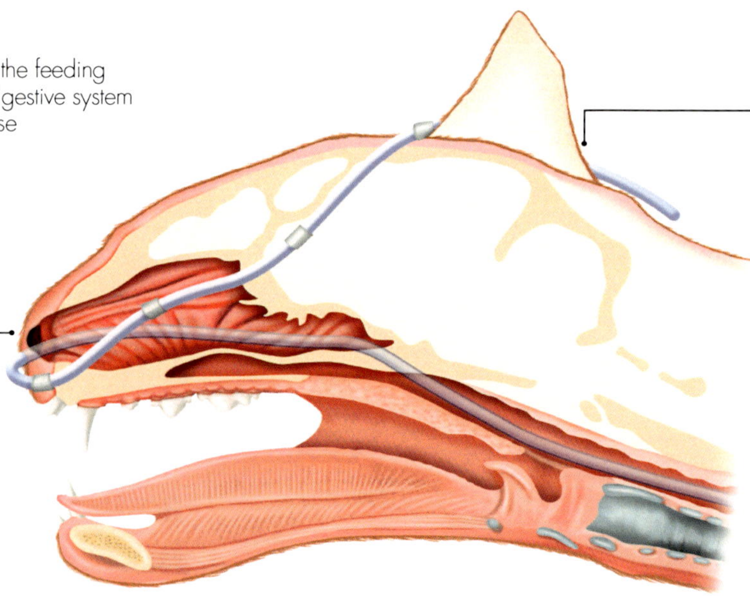

Advantages

- Simple procedure.

Disadvantages

- Requires an Elizabethan collar.
- Is uncomfortable for the cat.
- Can only be left for 6 days.

67 Collection of cerebrospinal fluid

Atlantooccipital puncture

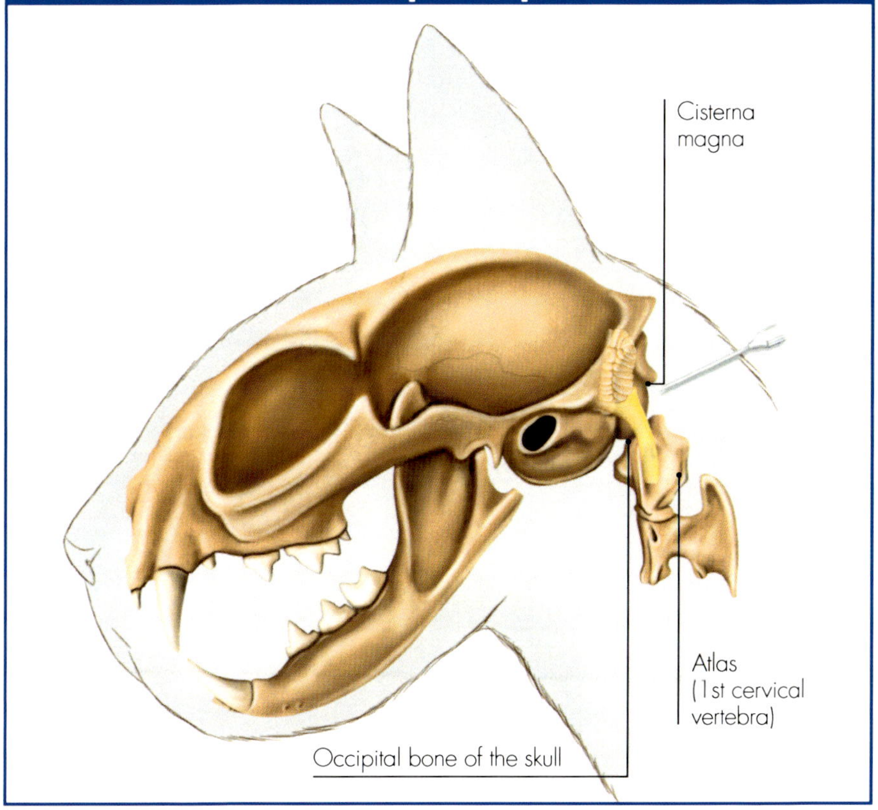

CSF is a colourless fluid which is distributed around the brain and spinal cord.
On occasions, its analysis is necessary to reach a precise diagnosis of the patient's disease: neurological processes of the central nervous system, bacterial infections or infectious diseases.

Technique for CSF collection

- The cat will be anaesthetised, since it must remain completely immobile during the procedure.
- CSF can be collected by means of an atlantooccipital puncture or lumbar puncture (between L5-L6 and L6-L7).

Lumbar puncture

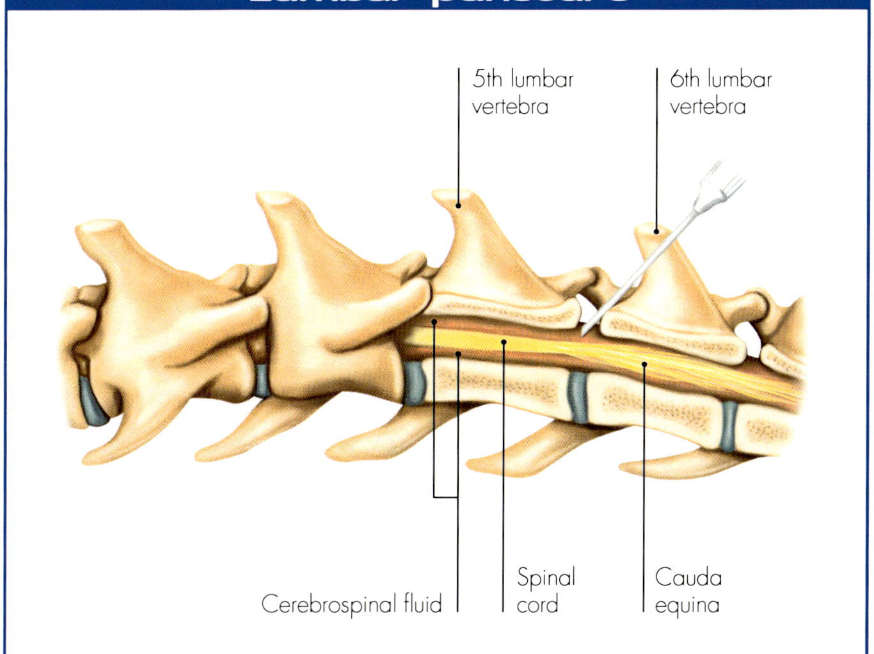

CSF analyses and cultures determine its cellular composition, biochemical characteristics and the possible presence of infectious agents.

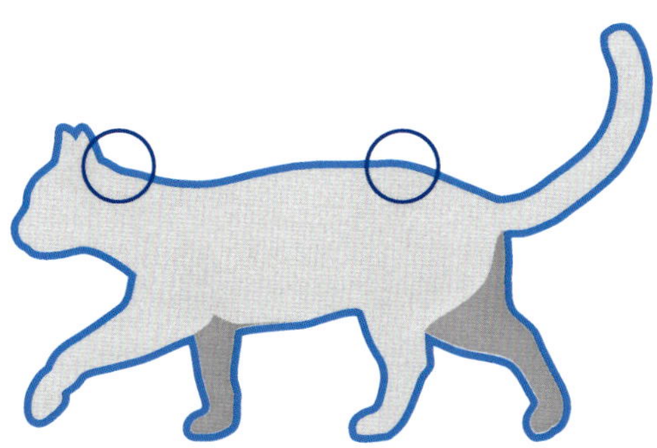

68 How to administer drugs

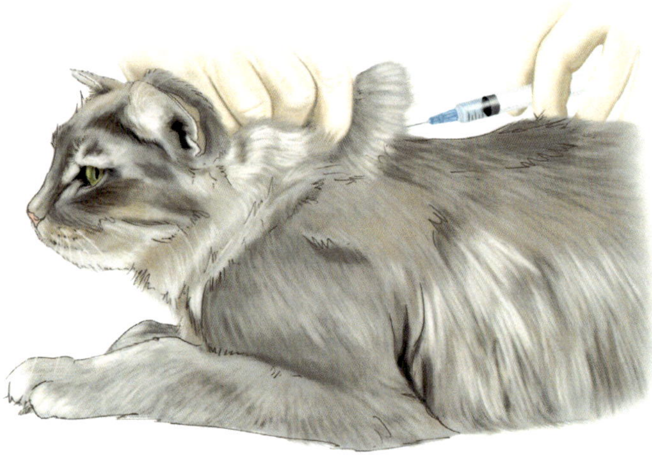

Subcutaneous injection

Eye drops

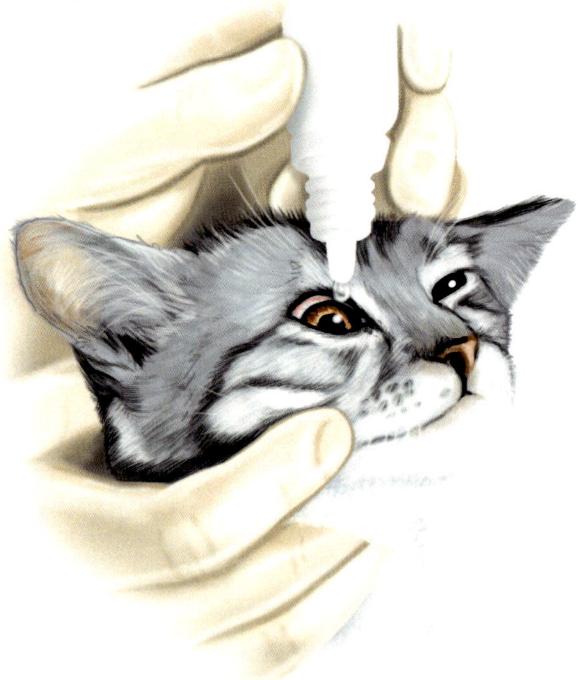

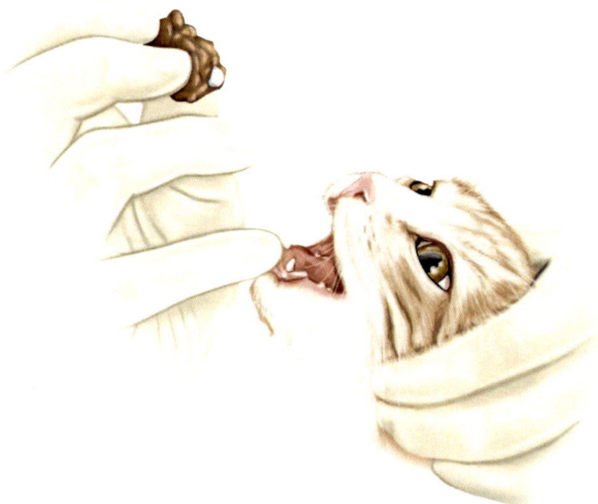

Drugs should never be mixed with the cat's usual food, as the cat would hate it from that moment on.

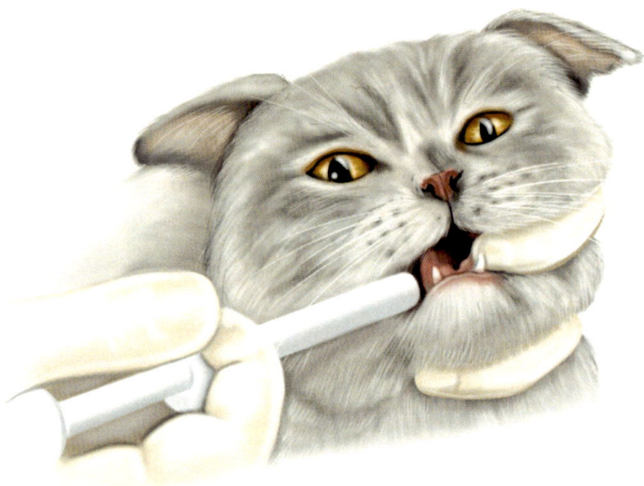

Administration of drugs by oral route

- The pill can be wrapped in meat, bread or butter to hide its taste.
- Water should always be given with a syringe immediately after administering drugs such as doxycycline or clyndamycin.
- The pills can be crushed and administered with water or sweet milk (if the veterinary surgeon considers it necessary).
- It is possible to use a pill gun instead of a syringe.

69 Postures and expressions in cats

Aggressive postures in cats

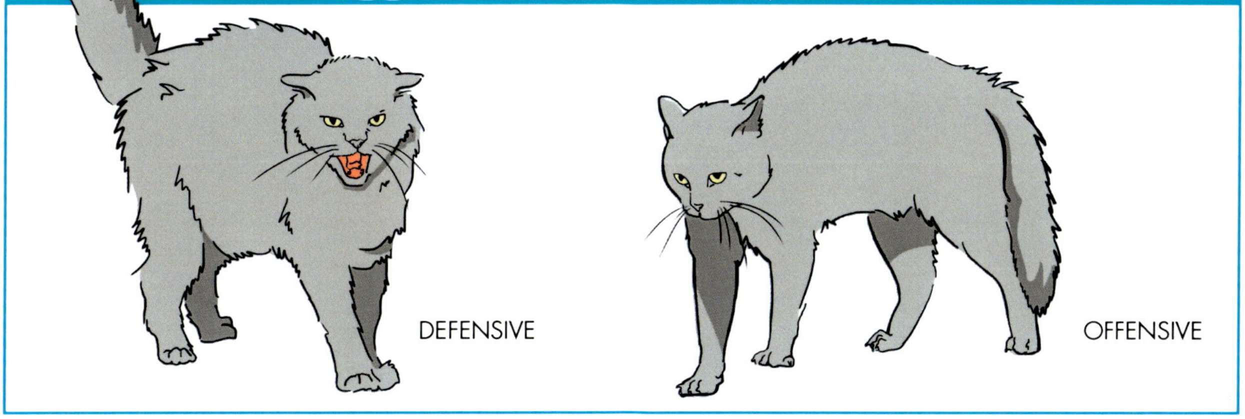

Usual postures in cats

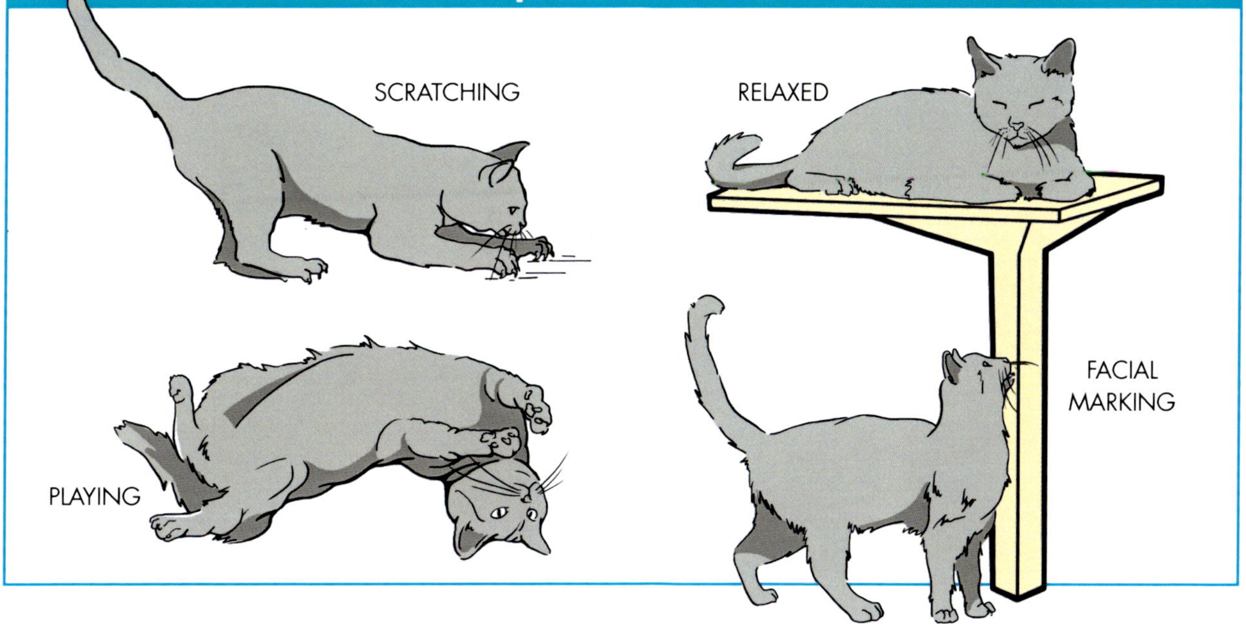

Expressions of pain

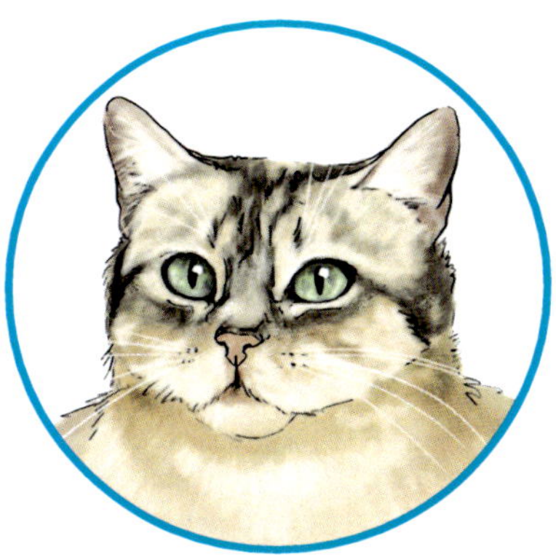

ABSENCE OF PAIN (round eyes)

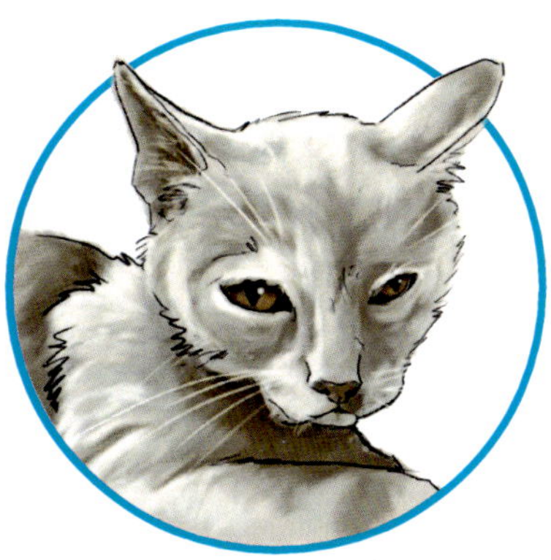

MODERATE PAIN (eyes partially closed)

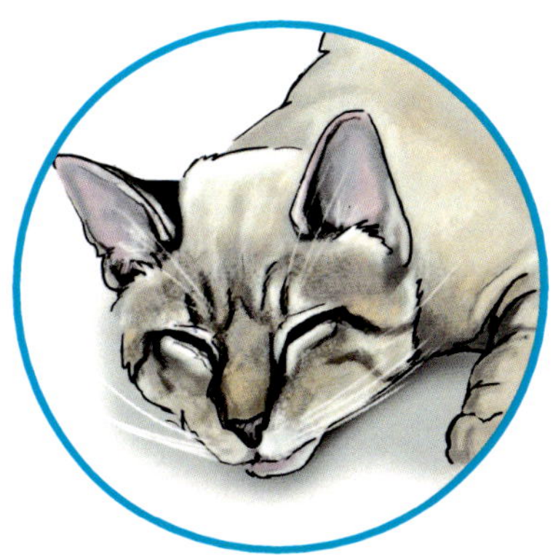

INTENSE PAIN (eyes mostly closed)

70 Neonate management

After birth, the best thing to do is to let the mother take care of her offspring. If she does not have a maternal instinct, we should immediately intervene: clear the airways and actively dry the kittens to stimulate respiration. After 24 hours, the kittens may be held with care to see their sex and ensure they are in good health. They should stay at home in a quiet place with an appropriate temperature, with their food and water bowls close to the nest.

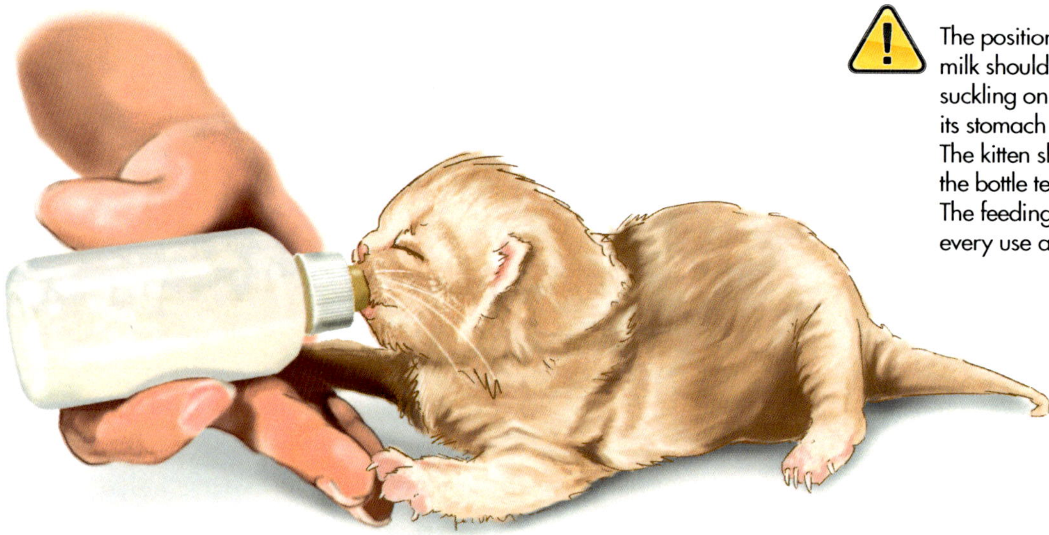

The position of the kitten when ingesting milk should be that adopted naturally when suckling on its mother, that is to say, lying on its stomach with the head stretched.
The kitten should be able to put its forelimbs on the bottle teat or on the carer's hands.
The feeding bottle should be washed after every use and sterilised at least once a day.

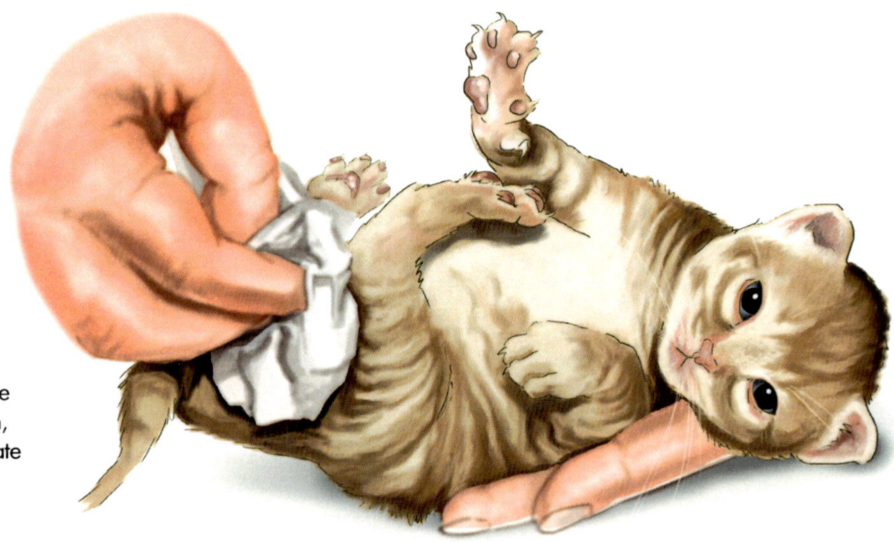

During the first 3-4 weeks of life, a gentle massage should be performed on the perianal area with a warm, damp cotton bud to stimulate micturition and defecation.

Orphaned kitten care

- Warm and constant ambient temperature (use of lamps, hot water bottles, blankets, etc.):
  - 1st week: 30-32 °C.
  - 2nd week: 26-29 °C.
  - From the 3rd week: 21-24 °C.
- Clean, comfortable place, with no air currents (e.g. box with a minimum height of 15 cm, with a towel or blanket).
- Feeding: special formula for kittens, warm (35-38 °C), administered every 2-3 hours during the first weeks of life by means of special feeding bottles or syringes (attached to a teat to prevent them from aspirating the milk).